Pediatrics

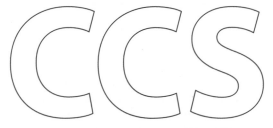

Correlations and **C**linical **S**cenarios

Pediatrics

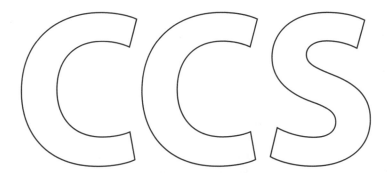

Correlations and Clinical Scenarios

Elizabeth V. August, MD
Chief Medical Officer of Bergen County
Riverside Medical and Pediatric Group
Hackensack, New Jersey

Niket Sonpal, MD
Assistant Clinical Professor of Medicine
Touro College of Medicine
New York, New York

St. Georges University School of Medicine
Assistant Clinical Professor of Medicine

Department of Gastroenterology
Lenox Hill Hospital
Northshore-LIJ Health System
New York, New York

Series Editor
Conrad Fischer, MD
Residency Program Director, Department of Medicine
Brookdale University Hospital Medical Center
Brooklyn, New York

Associate Professor of Physiology, Pharmacology and Medicine
Touro College of Medicine
New York, New York

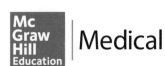 Medical

New York   Chicago   San Francisco   Athens   London   Madrid
Mexico City   Milan   New Delhi   Singapore   Sydney   Toronto

Correlations and Clinical Scenarios: Pediatrics

1 2 3 4 5 6 7 8 9 0   CTP/CTP   21 20 19 18 17 16

ISBN 978-0-07-181889-6
MHID 0-07-181889-8

This book was set in Arno Pro by Thomson Digital.
The editor was Regina Y. Brown.
The production supervisor was Catherine H. Saggese.
Project management was provided by Sarita Yadav, Thomson Digital.
China Translation & Printing Services was the printer and binder.
This book is printed on acid-free paper.

Library of Congress Cataloging-in-Publication Data

August, Elizabeth V., author.
  Correlations and clinical scenarios. Pediatrics / Elizabeth V. August, Niket Sonpal.
   p. ; cm.
  Pediatrics
  Includes bibliographical references and index.
  ISBN 978-0-07-181889-6 (pbk. : alk. paper)—ISBN 0-07-181889-8 (pbk : alk. paper)
  I. Sonpal, Niket, author. II. Title. III. Title: Pediatrics.
  [DNLM: 1. Pediatrics—Case Reports. 2. Pediatrics—Examination Questions.
3. Diagnosis, Differential—Case Reports. 4. Diagnosis, Differential—Examination
Questions. 5. Diagnostic Techniques and Procedures—Case Reports. 6. Diagnostic
Techniques and Procedures—Examination Questions. WS 18.2]
  RJ48.2
  618.920076—dc23
                                                                              2015006106

CONTENTS

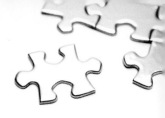

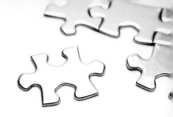

HOW TO USE THIS BOOK

The primary purpose of this book is to coach you in the precise sequence through time to manage the computerized case simulation (CCS) portion of the step 3 exam, specifically for questions pertaining to the specialty of Pediatrics. You will find directions on moving the clock forward in time and the specific sequence in which each test or treatment should be done in managing a patient. This will cover the order in which to give treatments, order tests, and how to respond to test results. All CCS-related instructions appear in RED TYPE.

If you have never seen a particular case, this book is especially for you. It never has statements about "using your judgment" because you basically do not have any in these areas. We have made a cookbook that says "Do this, do that, do this." We do not consider the term "cookbook" to be inappropriate in this case.

You need to learn the basics of pediatrics. Less than ten percent of physicians are in this specialty, but the other 90% need to have at least a working knowledge of it.

This book will prepare you for multiple-choice questions, which comprise the majority of the exam, as well as the computerized clinical case simulations and the new basic science foundations that have just been added to the exam.

USMLE Step 3 or COMLEX Part 3 is the last phase in getting your license. Most of you are in residency and have no time to study. Here is how to best use this book.

First read about the disease or subspecialty in any standard text book. We personally suggest either *Master the Boards Step 3* book (Conrad Fischer) or the *Current Medical Diagnosis and Treatment book.*

The cases in this book are meant to enhance your understanding of the subject. All initial case presentations and their continuing scenarios appear in yellow boxes. There are also hundreds of new multiple-choice questions that are not in anyone's Q bank.

Every single case has related basic science foundations (which appear in blue boxes), so you will get a solid grasp of these simply by following along in the case. You do not have to consult any of your old step 1 books or basic science texts. The basic science correlates should be painless. You need not search for extra information. Just learn what we have selected in these chapters.

We always wanted to write something specifically for CCS. This is it. Because new test changes are frightening and the basic science questions are new for step 3, we made one book to cover both the simulations and the basic science.

Elizabeth V. August, MD
Niket Sonpal, MD
Conrad Fischer, MD

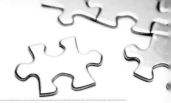

CHAPTER 1

NEWBORN MANAGEMENT

CASE 1: Heathy Newborn

Setting: *Hospital*

CC: *"I was just born."*

Vitals: *HR, 150 beats/min; RR, 30 breaths/min*

HPI: *Patient was born seconds ago to a 26-year-old G_1P_0 at 39 weeks' gestation. The mother had no medical problems and no gestational complications. The patient was born via normal spontaneous vaginal delivery (NSVD). The patient is screaming and crying.*

Physical Exam:
- *Gen: awake, crying, moving all limbs*
- *Head: No hematoma, open fontanels*
- *Eyes: + Red reflex*
- *Clavicles: Normal clavicles, no trauma noted*
- *CVS: S_1S_2 + tachycardia, no murmurs, rubs, gallops (no m/r/g)*
- *Lungs: Clear to auscultation bilaterally (CTA b/l)*
- *Abdomen: Soft, nontender, nondistended*
- *Rectum: Passage of meconium*
- *Genitalia: Penis, passage of urine, testicles descended bilaterally*
- *Spine: Straight, no patches of hair or spina bifida*
- *Hips: Negative Barlow and Ortolani*
- *Neurological: + Sucking reflex, + Moro reflex, + rooting reflex*
- *Skin: Pink centrally with blue tint noted in the extremities*

Which of the following is this baby's APGAR score?

a. 2 **d.** 8
b. 4 **e.** 9
c. 6

Answer e. 9

APGAR is a measure of how the baby is doing. It is based on the following scoring system.

APGAR Scoring System

	0 Points	1 Point	2 Points
Appearance	Pale blue	Pink body, blue extremities	Pink all over
Pulse	None	Less than 100	More than 100
Grimace (when stimulating child)	No response	Facial movement	Trying to pull away or crying
Activity	Limp	Flexion in arms and legs	Active movement
Respirations	None	Slow, irregular	Crying

Most babies only ever achieve a 9 because the skin tone almost always is pink centrally with bluish tinge in the extremities (acrocyanosis).

APGAR scores are done at 1 minute and 5 minutes after birth. The 1-minute score is based on how the baby was doing in utero, and the 5-minute score is how well the baby is responding to the resuscitative treatments or the environment.

In newborns, blood pressure is not routinely checked. Heart rate, respiratory rate, temperature, and weight are most often checked.

Range of normal vital sigs in newborns:
• Heart rate: 120 to 160 beats/min
• Respiratory rate: 30 to 50 breaths/min

After the baby is born, which of the following is the next step in the management of this patient?

a. Draw a CBC and blood cultures

b. Put erythromycin ointment in the patient's eyes

c. Do a blood glucose

d. Give hepatitis vaccination

Answer b. Put erythromycin ointment in the patient's eyes.

Erythromycin ointment should be put in the eyes of the newborn within 1 hour of birth. If the patient was shaky or had a an elevated temperature, the blood sugar, complete blood count (CBC), and blood cultures could be done. These tests are not routinely done in newborns. Hepatitis vaccination is not given within minutes of birth. The vitamin K injection is given within minutes of birth.

Mechanism of erythromycin
- Binds 50S subunit of ribosome
- Blocks translation of RNA
- Blocks protein production in bacteria

Gonorrhea
- Gram-negative diplococcus
- "Fastidious" = picky eaters!
- Only eats candy (glucose)
- Chocolate agar and 5% CO_2 growth
- Has "pili," which is a penis-like grappling hook that allows attachment to tissues

Pharmacokinetics of erythromycin
- Demethylation in liver
- Cytochrome P450 system
- Excretion through bile

Vitamin K is given to prevent hemorrhagic disease of the newborn.

For which of the following factors is vitamin K needed?

a. I

b. II

c. III

d. VI

e. V

Answer b. II

Vitamin K–dependent bleeding factors are factors II, VII, IX, and X. Newborns are given vitamin K at birth to prevent bleeding caused by vitamin deficiency. Breast milk does not provide adequate amounts. Without vitamin K, the baby may start to bleed intracranially or from the gastrointestinal tract, umbilical cord, nose, or circumcision site.

Mechanism of vitamin K
- Gamma carboxylation
- Adds carboxyl group to glutamate
- Formula has 100 times more vitamin K than human milk

Move the clock forward 1 hour.

The patient continues to do well and is crying intermittently. The mother would like to breastfeed the baby.

Which of the following is a contraindication to breastfeeding the newborn?

a. The mother had spinal anesthesia

b. The mother is positive for hepatitis B surface antibody

c. The mother has HIV

d. The mother has erythema of the breast

Answer c. The mother has HIV.

There are few absolute contraindications to breastfeeding. Maternal HIV and tuberculosis are the strongest absolute contraindications. Maternal herpes infection of the nipple is also a contraindication.

Anesthesia and pain medications are not contraindications to breastfeeding. Smoking and alcohol are relative contraindications, meaning that women should not smoke and drink and then breastfeed. If a woman chooses to smoke or drink alcohol, the milk should be expressed for a time before breastfeeding again. Mothers should be encouraged to not smoke, drink, or use drugs while pregnant or breastfeeding. If the patient has the hepatitis B surface antigen, it is not a contraindication to breastfeeding. Breastfeeding transmits as much HIV as passing through the birth canal.

Move the clock forward 1 hour.

The mother's hepatitis status is unknown. Blood is drawn for the hepatitis panel, and it returns that she is hepatitis B surface antigen positive.

Which of the following is the next step in the management of this patient?

a. Hepatitis B vaccination

b. Hepatitis immunoglobulin

c. Hepatitis immunoglobulin and hepatitis B vaccination

d. Quarantine the child and administer hepatitis B vaccine, hepatitis B immunoglobulin, and interferon

Answer c. Hepatitis B immunoglobulin and hepatitis B vaccination

All newborns will receive the hepatitis B vaccination before discharge from the hospital. Administration of the hepatitis immunoglobulins alone is insufficient.

Quarantining a child is unnecessary. It is unknown if the child had hepatitis B, and treatment would be unwarranted at this point.

HbcAg = hepatitis B core antigen
HbeAb = hepatitis B "e" antigen
BOTH are present during an active infection.

Mechanism of hepatitis B vaccine
• It is protein only.
• There is nothing "live" at all in hepatitis B vaccine.
• Recombinant production of surface antigen protein from yeast
• Surface antigen protein has no potential to initiate infection.

Move the clock forward 1 day.

Setting: *Hospital*
The mother states that the baby is latching onto the breast well and seems to be crying from hunger every 2 to 3 hours. The infant has had two or three bowel movements that are a greenish-yellow color.

Which of the following is NOT mandatory before discharge?

a. Newborn screening

b. Circumcision

c. Hearing test

Answer b. Circumcision

Circumcision is not required by any state. However, all states do require both the newborn screening and the hearing test. Hearing is needed for normal language development. If the patient is deaf or cannot hear normally, then there may be speech delay and behavioral changes in the child. Newborns are screened for brainstem responses to the sounds that are emitted from the apparatus. Since the implementation of newborn hearing screening, the average age of confirmation of deafness has dropped from 2 years old to 2 to 3 months.

Newborn screening is a mandatory blood test that is done to detect hormonal changes and inborn errors of metabolism. The tests are required by the state, but each individual state will have different requirements. More than 40 genetic tests are done in the newborn screening.

The patient was discharged healthy at 2 days of life. The patient's mother is to follow up with the primary care physician in 2 days.

CASE 2: Neonatal Jaundice

Setting: *Hospital*

CC: *"My baby looks yellow."*

Vitals: *HR, 120 beats/min; RR, 20 breaths/min; birth weight: 7lb, 6 oz; today's weight: 6 lb, 12 oz*

HPI: *The mother states that the baby has been latching onto the breast well, sucking well, and is crying every 2 or 3 hours. The infant has been urinating often and had 2 stools this morning. The baby is currently 2 days old. The mother states that she feels that the child is yellow in color. The mother is a G_1P_0 with no gestational complications during pregnancy. The mother was group B streptococcus (GBS) negative.*

Physical Exam:
- *Gen: Awake, alert*
- *Head: Asymmetric; small collection on top of head that does not cross the suture lines*
- *Clavicles: Normal, no birth trauma noted*
- *CVS: S_1S_2+, tachycardia, no m/r/g*
- *Lungs: CTA b/l*
- *Abdomen: Soft, NT, ND, +BS*
- *Skin: Slight yellowing of the skin*

Which of the following is the next step in the management of this patient?

a. Bilirubin levels

b. CBC and blood cultures

c. Start phototherapy

d. Exchange transfusion

Answer a. Bilirubin levels

This patient seems to be slightly jaundiced. The next step in the management of a jaundiced baby is to order a bilirubin level; blood type and screen; and if the patient is at risk for in infection (e.g., the mother was GBS positive without adequate treatment during delivery), then a CBC or blood cultures. Treatment with phototherapy and exchange transfusion is too early at this point. All babies will become slightly jaundiced after birth, but if it increases to a dangerous level, then phototherapy or exchange transfusion may be considered.

Newborns normally lose weight in the first week of life. It should NEVER be more than 10%.

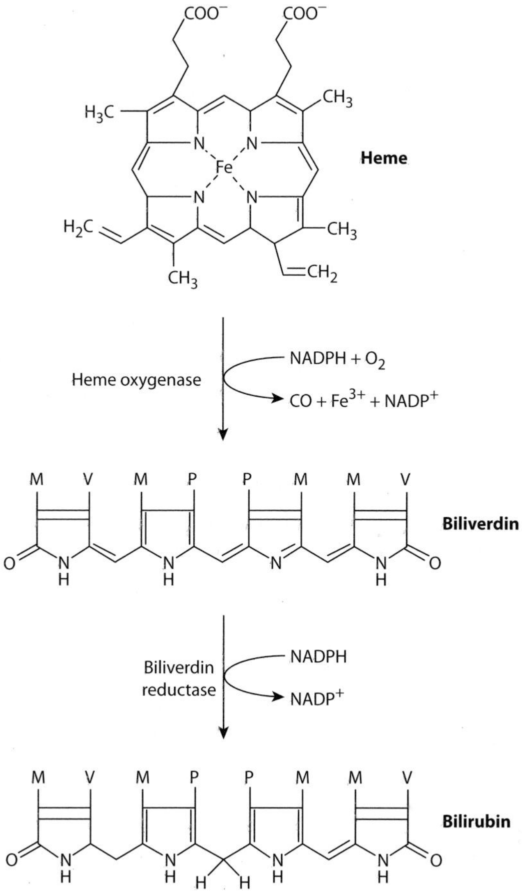

Figure 1-1. Molecular breakdown of hemoglobin to bilirubin. (Reproduced with permission from Barrett KE, et al. Chapter 28. Transport & metabolic functions of the liver. In: Barrett KE, et al., eds. *Ganong's Review of Medical Physiology.* 24th ed. New York, NY: McGraw-Hill; 2012. Figure 28-4.)

Biochemical pathway of bilirubin production
- Bilirubin is a byproduct of heme breakdown.
- Porphyrin of heme broken down by heme oxygenase (Figure 1-1)
- Biliverdin converted in the macrophage to bilirubin

Bilirubin level was drawn and returns at 12 mg/dL. The patient and her mother have the same blood type, O+.

Which of the following is the next step in the management of this patient?

a. Start phototherapy

b. Start exchange transfusion

c. Start supplementation with formula

d. This is a normal level; there is no need for intervention

Answer c. Start supplementation with formula

The test results need to be interpreted with a graph. Generally speaking, it is the hours of life versus the bilirubin level. If there is noticeable jaundice in the first day of life, it is pathological, and aggressive diagnosis and treatment should be initiated. If the patient is found to be in the low-intermediate risk zone or high-intermediate risk zone, then supplementation should be started. One of the most common reasons for jaundice is breast milk jaundice. Breast milk jaundice occurs when the patient is a little dehydrated because there is not enough milk produced. Generally, supplementation with formula will only need to be done for about 1 week. After the milk comes in, most patients no longer need to supplement. However, after supplementation starts, the patient's bilirubin level should be checked to assure that the bilirubin level is decreasing (Figure 1-2).

Which of the following is the most likely reason for this patient to have jaundice?

a. ABO incompatibility

b. Cephalohematoma

c. Breastfeeding jaundice

d. G6PD

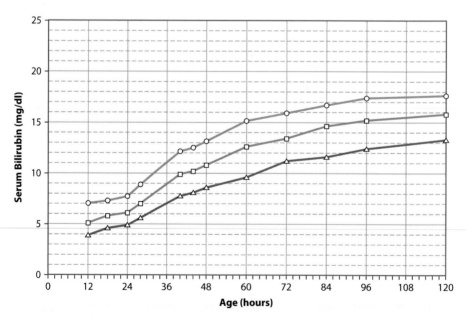

Figure 1-2. Nomogram for newborn bilirubin. (*Source:* http://www.fda.gov/ohrms/dockets/ac/03/slides/3965OPH1_01_Bhutani_files/slide0240_image084.gif.)

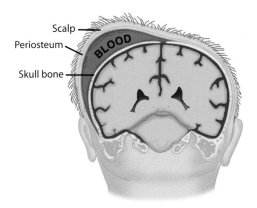

Scalp

Periosteum

BLOOD

Skull bone

Figure 1-3. Cephalohematoma. (Reproduced with permission from Diseases and injuries of the fetus and newborn. In: Cunningham FG, et al., eds. *Williams Obstetrics*. 23rd ed. New York, NY: McGraw-Hill; 2010.)

Answer b. Cephalohematoma

Cephalohematoma is a hemorrhage collection on the outside of the skull (Figure 1-3). Cephalohematoma occurs during the birth process and is a common complication of vacuum-assisted deliveries. This collection of blood needs to be reabsorbed by the body, and if present in a newborn, it almost always causes jaundice.

Cephalohematoma causes jaundice secondary to a nonhemolytic increase in bilirubin production. ABO incompatibility is a common reason for jaundice among patients. This generally occurs in mothers with blood type O. Hemolysis can range from mild to severe depending on the amount of antibody the mother has produced. The Coombs test result will be positive in these patients. G6PD deficiency is a common red blood cell (RBC) enzyme deficiency that can cause hemolysis. It is an X-linked disorder that should be specifically tested for if results for the more common causes are negative. Breastfeeding jaundice is the most common type of jaundice in the first week of life. It is secondary to decreased milk production during this time.

Risk factors for hyperbilirubinemia
- Jaundice in first 24 hours of life
- ABO incompatibility
- Cephalohematoma
- Previous sibling needing phototherapy
- Exclusive breastfeeding

Direct Coombs test
- Put antibodies against Fc portions of IgG.
- Look for agglutination.

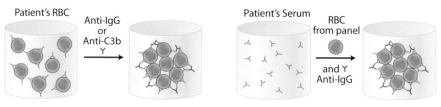

Figure 1-4. Indirect Coombs test. (Reproduced with permission from Bunn H. Acquired hemolytic anemias. In: Bunn H, Aster JC, eds. *Pathophysiology of Blood Disorders*. New York, NY: McGraw-Hill; 2011.)

Indirect Coombs test
- Put RBCs in with plasma.
- Antibodies, if present, attach to RBCs.
- Add IgG antibodies to the Fc portions of IgG attached to RBCs.
- If warm antibodies are present, clumping of cells will occur (Figure 1-4).

G6PD
- Loss of production of glutathione reductase
- Insufficient reducing capacity of RBCs
- Oxidant stress precipitate RBC hemoglobin
- Precipitated RBC hemoglobin is Heinz bodies

The mother started to supplement the baby with formula to help increase excretion of the bilirubin. The bilirubin level increased to 15 mg/dL. The baby is acting normal but appears to be more yellow in color.

Which of the following is the next step in the management of this patient?

a. Intravenous (IV) hydration

b. Increase oral supplementation

c. Start phototherapy

d. Start exchange transfusion

Answer c. Start phototherapy

With cephalohematoma, increasing bilirubin levels put the patient at increased risk for bilirubin toxicity or kernicterus. Bilirubin deposition in neurons is the most dangerous complication of jaundice. Kernicterus can lead to irreversible brain damage that causes cerebral palsy and hearing difficulties.

To try to prevent this damage from occurring, treatment of the hyperbilirubinemia should occur. The two treatments include phototherapy and exchange transfusion. Each of these is based on a nomogram. Phototherapy is safe and noninvasive. The patient is placed under ultraviolet light, and the bilirubin is checked every 6 to 8 hours to ensure that that level is decreasing. If an exchange transfusion is needed, it is a medical emergency. It is invasive and risky, but luckily, it is not needed often now that phototherapy is used routinely.

Mechanism of kernicterus
- Bilirubin-induced brain dysfunction
- Bilirubin binds phospholipids of neurons
- Permanent damage
- Hearing loss

Elimination of bilirubin through stool
- Released with bile through the bile duct to the bowel
- Glucuronic acid removed by bacteria in bowel
- Conversion to stercobilin
- Stercobilin gives stool brown color and is eliminated

CASE 3: Neonatal Hypoglycemia

Setting: *Hospital*

CC: *"My baby is shaky."*

Vitals: *HR, 130 beats/min; RR, 25 breaths/min*

HPI: *A baby boy born 30 minutes ago is shaky and irritable. The baby was born to a G_1P_0 woman with diet-controlled gestational diabetes at 39 weeks. The patient's APGAR scores were 9 of 10 at 1 and 5 minutes.*

Physical Exam:
- *Gen: Awake, alert, shaky, crying*
- *CVS: S_1S_2+ Tachycardia, no m/r/b*
- *Lungs: CTA b/l*
- *Abd: Soft +BS*
- *Ext: No cyanosis*

Which of the following is the next step in the management of this patient?

a. Drug screening   **c.** CBC
b. Blood glucose

Answer b. Blood glucose

Blood glucose is done before a CBC and drug screen because it will yield the quickest results. Blood glucose is done at the bedside with a heel stick, and results return within minutes. A CBC and drug screen may be done, but blood glucose is always the first step. Blood glucose is usually 15 mg/dL less than the mothers. However, after the patient is born, there is a quick drop in blood glucose. Glucose often drops as low as 30 in normal, healthy, term infants within 1 or 2 hours of life. Hypoglycemia in a term neonate is defined as a blood glucose level less than 40 mg/dL after feeding.

Glucose drops rapidly after birth. It may drop as low as 30 mg/dL.
Hypoglycemia = after feeding <40 mg/dL
Glucose stabilizes after 3 hours at around 45 mg/dL.

Blood glucose returns at 40 mg/dL after breastfeeding.

Which of the following mechanisms caused this patient's hypoglycemia?

a. Maternal hypoglycemia

b. Maternal hyperinsulinemia

c. Decreased glycogen storage in the fetus

d. Fetal hyperglycemia in utero

Answer d. Fetal hyperglycemia in utero

Infants of diabetic mothers (IDMs) are at significant risk for hypoglycemia. Risk factors for hypoglycemia include IDM, intrauterine growth restriction (IUGR), Beckwidth-Wiedemann syndrome, inborn errors of metabolism, stress, birth trauma, infections, and hypoxia. IDMs have hypoglycemia secondary to an increase in the fetal insulin secondary to hyperglycemia while the patient was in utero. The fetus is surrounded by extra glucose for 9 months, causing there to be an excessive amount of glycogen storage and hyperinsulinemia in the fetus. However, when the infant is suddenly removed from all of the extra sugar in the environment, the high levels of insulin the baby was producing now make the baby hypoglycemic. Decreased glycogen storage in the fetus occurs in IUGR. The excess insulin drives all.

Biochemistry of insulin
- Insulin uses tyrosine kinase receptor in most tissues.
- Insulin activates lipoprotein lipase (LPL).
- LPL removes glucose from blood and puts in storage at fat.
- Insulin puts glucose in storage in liver as glycogen.
- Neural tissue and exercising muscle do not need insulin.
- Glucose stored as fat can only come out as fat.

Risk factors for hypoglycemia
- IDMs
- IUGR
- Inborn errors of metabolism
- Galactosemia
- Stress
- Birth trauma
- Asphyxia
- Sepsis

Which of the following is the treatment of this patient?

a. Feed the baby

b. Start D5W (dextrose 5% in water)

c. Start D10W (dextrose 10% in water)

Answer a. Feed the baby.

Infants who are hypoglycemic should be fed as long as they are alert. Infants often are alert and crying despite the hypoglycemia. If the infant is lethargic, then starting D10W would be indicated.

> *Despite the low blood sugar, the patient was crying and was given formula. After ingesting the formula, the patient's blood sugar increased. It was checked several times throughout the nursery stay and remained normal.*

CASE 4: **Respiratory Distress in the Newborn**

Setting: *Hospital*

CC: *"My baby is not breathing well."*

Vitals: *HR, 145 beats/min; RR, 45 breaths/min*

HPI: *The patient was born via cesarean section 1 hour ago to a G_1P_0 mother with no gestational complications at 39 weeks. The mother had routine prenatal care and no medical problems during her pregnancy. The mother states that patient appears to not be breathing well.*

Physical Exam:
- *Gen: Awake and alert*
- *Head: NC, no cephalohematoma*
- *Chest: Ribs can be seen between breaths, intercostal retractions*
- *Lungs: Crackles bilaterally*
- *CVS: S_1S_2+ tachycardia, no m/r/g*
- *Abd: Soft, NT, ND, +BS*
- *Ext: No cyanosis noted*

Which of the following is the next step in the management of this patient?

a. Chest radiography

b. Nasogastric tube placement

c. Administration of surfactant

d. CBC, CMP, and blood cultures

Answer a. Chest radiography

Chest radiography (CXR), pulse oxygenation, or arterial blood gas (ABG) are the first steps in the management of ANY patient with respiratory distress. ABG, pulse oxygenation (pulse ox), and CXR all help establish that the patient is in respiratory distress, determine the severity of it, and lead to possible etiologies of the distress. CBC, CMP, and blood cultures would be done if the distress was caused by a possible infection. Administration of surfactant would be done if the infant was premature. Nasogastric tube placement may be done if the respiratory distress started after the first feeding.

Respiratory distress = CXR, ABG, and pulse ox

Move the clock forward 20 minutes.

The CXR returns with perihilar streaking. Pulse ox is 89%.

Which of the following is the most likely diagnosis?

a. Transient tachypnea of the newborn (TTN)

b. Meconium aspiration

c. Spontaneous pneumothorax

d. Pneumonia

e. Hyaline membrane disease of the newborn

f. Diaphragmatic hernia

Answer a. Transient tachypnea of the newborn (TTN)

The patient did not have a chance to go through the birth canal. When infants do not go through the birth canal or do so but quickly, they do not have the chance to have their lungs squeezed and get rid of all the amniotic fluid that was previously there. The infant's lungs and body will reabsorb the fluid in 24 to 48 hours.

Respiratory Disease in Newborn

Disease	History	CXR Finding
TTN	Born via cesarean delivery or quick stage 2 of labor (quick passage through the birth canal)	Perihilar streaking
Meconium aspiration	In utero distress or stressed baby	Irregular infiltrates, hyperexpansion, or lobar pneumonia
Spontaneous pneumothorax	Respiratory distress from birth; decreased breath sounds on affected side	Area of air surrounding the outside of lung
Pneumonia	Fever, tachycardia, tachypnea	Lobar consolidation
Hyaline membrane disease	Premature infants with respiratory distress	Hypoexpansion; air bronchograms
Diaphragmatic hernia	Respiratory distress since birth; bowel sounds in chest	Bowel in chest and small lung on affected side

On the test, they must give you a clue to which diagnosis it is!

What is the next step in the management of this patient?

a. Observation

b. Oxygen

c. IV ampicillin and gentamicin

d. Surfactant

e. Surgical intervention

f. Chest tube placement

Answer b. Oxygen

This infant's oxygen saturation is 89%, so oxygen needs to be administered. If the patient's oxygen saturation were above 95%, then observation would have been correct.

Treatment of Respiratory Disease of Newborn

Disease	Treatment
TTN	Observation or oxygen (depends on the oxygenation of the infant)
Meconium aspiration	
Spontaneous pneumothorax	Observation and oxygen administration, but if >30% pneumothorax, then chest tube or needle decompression is needed
Pneumonia	IV ampicillin and IV gentamicin
Hyaline membrane disease	Administration of surfactant
Diaphragmatic hernia	Surgical correction of the hernia

Why does hyperventilation RAISE the pO_2 (Figure 1-5)?
- Hyperventilation DECREASES pCO_2.
- Decreasing pCO_2 should INCREASE the paO_2 or amount of oxygen in blood.
- pCO_2 going from 40 to 20 should INCREASE the paO_2 to 125.
- This is why an 89% saturation with a respiratory rate of 65 breaths/min is so bad in this patient!

$$pAO_2 = 150 - \frac{pCO_2}{0.8}$$

Figure 1-5. A-a gradient. (Used with permission from Conrad Fischer.)

Move the clock forward 24 hours.

The patient's breathing is less labored, and he is no longer requiring oxygen. The patient should be discharged at 3 days of life.

Discharge timing as long as it is an uncomplicated stay:
NSVD = 2 days of life
Cesarean delivery = 3 days of life

CASE 5: Hyaline Membrane Disease

Setting: *ED*

CC: *"My baby was not supposed to come this early."*

Vitals: *HR, 150 beats/min; RR, 75 breaths/min*

HPI: *A mother rushes her baby into the emergency department (ED), stating that she just gave birth in the car. She was having severe cramps, but the baby was only at 29 weeks of gestational age. She did not think she could deliver the baby this early. The baby was born about 10 minutes ago. The mother is a 17-year-old G_1P_0 with minimal prenatal care.*

PE of baby:
- *Gen: Small, about 2.5 lb*
- *Head: Atraumatic, no cephalohematomas*
- *Chest: Intercostal retractions, tachypnea, grunting, nasal flaring, poor air movement*
- *CVS: S_1S_2+ tachycardia, no murmurs heard*
- *Ext: Cyanotic*

Which of the following is the next step in the management of this baby?

a. Administer oxygen

b. Chest radiography

c. ABG

d. Administer surfactant

Answer a. Administer oxygen

This baby is in severe respiratory distress. Although the patient needs chest radiography, ABG, and possibly surfactant, the baby needs oxygen the most. Severe respiratory distress means there is a respiratory rate greater than 30 breaths/min, grunting and intercostal retraction, and cyanosis in the extremities. Although all of the tests and administering the surfactant are correct, the first thing we do is to administer oxygen.

On the CCS: Order oxygen, intubation, CXR, and ABG all at the same time. On the CCS, respiratory distress in a premature infant is a circumstance when giving oxygen and ordering tests at the same time is appropriate because of the life-threatening nature of impending respiratory failure.

Which of the following could have prevented this?

a. Administration of ampicillin during labor

b. Prenatal vitamin usage

c. Antenatal steroid administration

d. Avoidance of illegal drugs during pregnancy

e. Influenza vaccine

Answer c. Antenatal steroid administration

If the patient had presented to labor and delivery at 29 weeks' gestation with severe contractions, steroids would have been given. Steroids are given to help increase the surfactant production over a 24- to 28-hour period. This has been proven to decrease infants' mortality rate. Prenatal vitamins are always recommended to help prevent neural tube defects.

Administration of ampicillin during labor will decrease the risk of the fetus developing GBS sepsis. This is done when screening culture of the cervix shows GBS.

Avoidance of illegal drugs during pregnancy is always recommended. However, cocaine specifically can cause placental abruption and premature delivery of the fetus.

> *Oxygen is being administered, and the CXR results return with diffuse atelectasis and ground-glass appearance.*

Which of the following is the next step in the management of this patient?

a. Administration of ampicillin and gentamicin

b. Administration of surfactant

c. Administration of corticosteroids

Answer b. Administration of surfactant

Patients who are thought to have hyaline membrane disease should be intubated as soon as possible for the administration of surfactant. Administration of ampicillin and gentamicin would be useful if the patient had pneumonia. Corticosteroids only are effective when given to the mother before the baby's birth. They do not help after the baby is born.

Mechanism of surfactant
• Surfactant separates water molecules
• Decreases surface tension of alveoli
• Increases the surface area of alveolus

Law of Laplace (Figure 1-6)
• Bigger alveoli have LESS surface tension.
• Smaller alveoli collapse MORE.

Small radius = big pressure of collapse

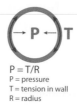

$P = T/R$
P = pressure
T = tension in wall
R = radius

Figure 1-6. Law of Laplace. (Used with permission from Conrad Fischer.)

Advance the clock 12 hours.

The patient still requires 30% oxygenation via ventilator. Physical exam findings are unchanged. The patient's lungs still sound coarse and have crackles bilaterally.

Which of the following is the next step in the management of this patient?

a. Repeat administration of surfactant   **c.** Administer IV antibiotics
b. Observe patient   **d.** Administer albuterol

Answer a. Repeat administration of surfactant

If the patient is still requires greater than 30% to 40% oxygen after administration of surfactant, up to three doses may be given. Albuterol and IV antibiotics are still not indicated. Oxygen administration should be kept to the minimum needed. Inspired oxygen levels above 50% can lead to lung fibrosis. If there is fibrosis, more positive pressure needs to be given to inflate the lung. If more positive pressure is needed to inflate the lung, then rupture of the lung, or barotrauma is more likely.

Mechanism of surfactant
• Surfactant literally gets in between the water molecules
• A phospholipid acts like soap to break bonds between water molecules
• Decreases the surface tension of water in the alveoli (Figure 1-7)

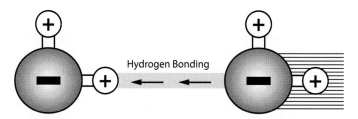

Hydrogen Bonding

Figure 1-7. Mechanism of surfactant. (Used with permission from Conrad Fischer.)

After two doses of surfactant, the baby is starting to breath better on his own and is switched to nasal continuous positive airway pressure.

CASE 6: Necrotizing Enterocolitis

Setting: *Hospital*

CC: *"My baby's stomach seems large."*

Vitals: *HR, 150 beats/min; RR, 40 breaths/min; T: 98.7°F*

HPI: *A 32-year-old woman with no past medical history gave birth to a baby boy 2 days ago at 31 weeks' gestational age. The patient was in preterm labor for 3 days and received corticosteroids to help mature the lungs. The baby has had an uneventful 2 days of life. This morning, his abdomen became enlarged. Heme-positive stool was expressed less than 1 hour ago.*

Physical Exam:
- *Gen: Awake, alert, crying*
- *CVS: S_1S_2+ Tachycardia*
- *Lungs: Clear bilaterally*
- *Abd: Generalized tenderness, abdominal distension is present*
- *Ext: No cyanosis noted*

Which of the following is the next step in the management of this baby?

a. Stop oral intake for the child (NPO)   **d.** CMP
b. Abdominal radiography   **e.** Administer oxygen
c. CBC

Answer a. Stop oral intake for the child (NPO)

The child may have the beginning signs of necrotizing enterocolitis (NEC). The major risk factor for NEC is prematurity. However, just because the patient has heme-positive stool and abdominal distension, it is not a confirmed diagnosis. In all cases of blood in the stool of a newborn, feeding should be stopped until a diagnosis is achieved. In NEC, feeding is contraindicated because it will lead to worsening of the disease. NEC is a pediatric emergency. Patients with NEC start to deteriorate quickly. They may start to have fluctuations in their body temperature, perforation of the intestines, apnea, and bradycardia. After a diagnosis is established, parenteral feeding should occur. Refeeding may start slowly after the radiographs have showed resolution.

Which of the following test is first to show a diagnosis?

a. CBC   **d.** Abdominal CT
b. CMP   **e.** Abdominal radiography
c. Blood cultures

Answer e. Abdominal radiography

On the CCS, the following orders should be placed on the initial screen: NPO, CBC, CMP, blood cultures, abdominal radiography, prothrombin time, and activated partial thromboplastin time.

Abdominal radiography is the test of choice because it will show pneumatosis intestinalis. These are air bubbles in the walls of the intestine in the infant. Only if the abdominal radiography is unequivocal will a CT then need to be done. Do not expose newborns to radiation unless it is ABSOLUTELY necessary. CBC, CMP, and blood cultures should all be done but will only prove that the infant has an infection. Small bowel obstruction is one of the few indications for abdominal radiography.

NEC symptoms:
- Feeding problems
- Vomiting
- Abdominal distension
- Abdominal tenderness
- Abdominal wall cellulitis

Distension + Heme in stool + Air in bowel on radiographs = NEC

NEC risk factors
- Prematurity (#1 risk factor because of low birth weight)
- Congenital heart disease
- Birth asphyxia

Pneumatosis intestinalis = air in the walls of the intestines

Interval History:
- *White blood cell (WBC) count: 25*
- *Hemoglobin: 13*
- *Hematocrit: 38*
- *Platelet count: 100,000*
- *Abdominal radiography shows pneumatosis intestinalis. No free air under the diaphragm (Figure 1-8).*

The patient continues to breathe on his own without any signs of apnea. His abdomen is still distended.

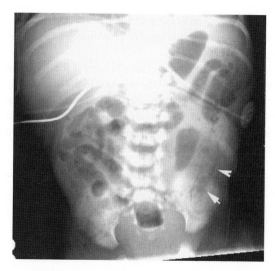

Figure 1-8. Pneumatosis intestinalis. (Reproduced with permission from Hackam DJ, et al. Pediatric surgery. In: Brunicardi F, et al., eds. *Schwartz's Principles of Surgery.* 10th ed. New York, NY: McGraw-Hill; 2014.)

Which of the following is the next step in the management of this patient?

a. IV ampicillin, gentamicin, and metronidazole

b. IV ciprofloxacin and metronidazole

c. Surgical intervention

d. Methylprednisolone

e. IV immunoglobulin

Answer a. IV ampicillin, gentamicin, and metronidazole

IV antibiotics should be administered because this patient's WBC count is elevated; the drugs of choice are ampicillin and gentamicin. Newborns and children should NEVER receive ciprofloxacin. Surgical intervention is not needed at this time because there are no signs of perforation. A nasogastric (NG) tube should be placed instead to help decompress the gut of this baby.

Steroids will only make potential immunocompromised worse. IV immunoglobulins would not be useful. The baby has maternal IgG that passed the placenta.

Mechanism of quinolone contraindication in children
- Bone and cartilage abnormalities
- Inhibition of osteoblasts
- Inhibition of chondroblasts

Prognosis:
- The mortality rate for NEC is 10%.
- Long-term outcomes depend on the amount of bowel lost.

Move clock forward 1 day.

Repeat abdominal radiography shows worsening of the pneumatosis intestinalis, small amounts of air under the diaphragm, and the NG tube in place.

What is the next step?

a. Continue to monitor the infant

b. Surgical intervention

c. Start mechanical ventilation

d. Add vancomycin

Answer b. Surgical intervention

Patients who have free air under the diaphragm need surgery. Free air under the diaphragm means that there has been a perforation in the intestines. This hole will leak bowel contents into the abdominal cavity and cause peritonitis. This is a surgical emergency. Starting mechanical ventilation at this point will not help. Changing his antibiotics may be indicated, but surgery is mandatory.

Air under diaphragm = perforation = surgery

Surgical indications
- Perforation (air under the diaphragm)
- Abdominal wall cellulitis
- Fixed dilated loop of bowel on multiple radiographs

The patient was sent to surgery with resolution of the perforation.

CASE 7: Congenital Malformation

Setting: *Hospital*

CC: *"What is that!?"*

Vitals: *HR, 150 beats/min; RR, 40 breaths/min*

HPI: *The patient was born minutes ago to a 26-year-old woman. The mother is a healthy woman who received routine prenatal care. The patient did not have any complications during pregnancy or labor and delivery. The mother was handed the baby, but there was a deformity present on his abdomen.*

Physical Exam:
- Gen: *Awake, crying; APGAR scores, 9, 9*
- Head: *NC, no cephalohematoma noted, sutures open*
- Eyes: *+ Red reflex bilaterally*
- Ears: *Patent*
- Mouth: *No cleft lip or cleft palate*
- CVS: S_1S_2+ *No murmurs heard*
- Lungs: *Clear*
- Abd: *Soft, midline opening with gastric contents found outside of abdominal wall; transparent sac surrounding abdominal contents.*
- Ext: *No abnormalities noted*

Which of the following is the diagnosis?

a. Diaphragmatic hernia

b. Omphalocele

c. Gastroschisis

d. Meckel diverticulum

e. Malrotation

f. Duodenal atresia

Answer b. Omphalocele

Congenital Malformations

Deformity	Description	Image (Figures 1-9 to 1-14)
Diaphragmatic hernia	Hole in the diaphragm; intestines go through hole and develop in the chest	

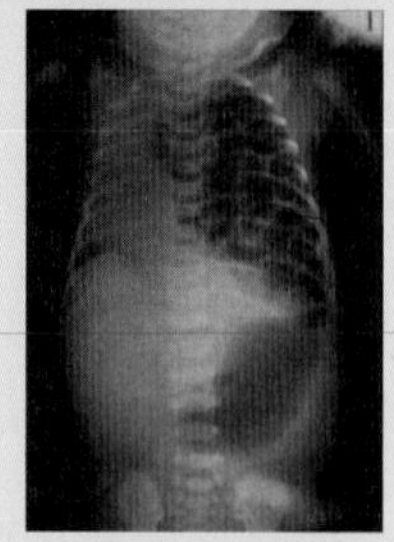

Figure 1-9. Diaphragmatic hernia. (Reproduced with permission from Ahern G, Brygel M. Exploring Essential Radiology. http://accesssurgery.mhmedical.com/ multimedia.aspx#tab=3.)

Omphalocele	Abdominal contents are outside of body with a sac around them	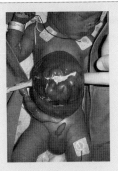 **Figure 1-10.** Omphalocele. (Reproduced with permission from Hackam DJ, et al. Pediatric surgery. In: Brunicardi F, et al., eds. *Schwartz's Principles of Surgery.* 10th ed. New York, NY: McGraw-Hill; 2014.)
Gastroschisis	Abdominal contents are outside of body without a sac around them	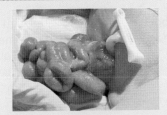 **Figure 1-11.** Gastroschisis. (Reproduced with permission from Hackam DJ, et al. Pediatric surgery. In: Brunicardi F, et al., eds. *Schwartz's Principles of Surgery.* 10th ed. New York, NY: McGraw-Hill; 2014.)
Meckel diverticulum	Stray area of gastric acid production within the gastrointestinal (GI) tract that often causes bleeding. (See more information in the GI section)	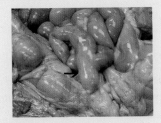 **Figure 1-12.** Meckel diverticulum. (Reproduced with permission from Kemp WL, Burns DK, Brown TG. Chapter 14. Gastrointestinal pathology. In: Kemp WL, Burns DK, Brown TG, eds. *Pathology*: The Big Picture. New York, NY: McGraw-Hill; 2008.)

(Continued)

Deformity	Description	Image
Malrotation	Bowel twisted around itself; causes bilious vomiting	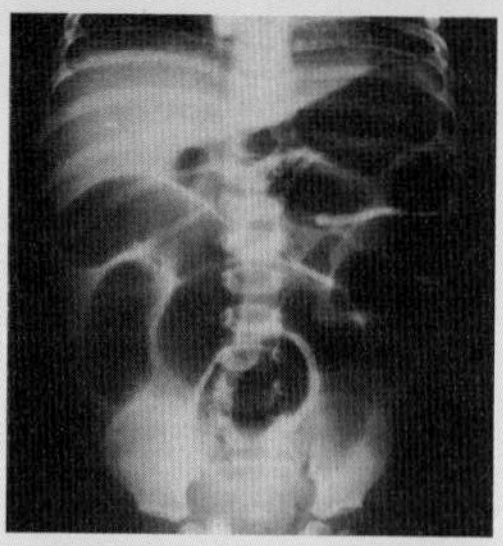 Figure 1-13. Malrotation. (Reproduced with permission from Kharbanda AB, Sawaya RD. Chapter 124. Acute abdominal pain in children. In: Tintinalli JE, et al., eds. *Tintinalli's Emergency Medicine*: A Comprehensive Study Guide. 7th ed. New York, NY: McGraw-Hill; 2011.)
Duodenal atresia	Associated with Down syndrome; no passage of air or gastric contents past the duodenum	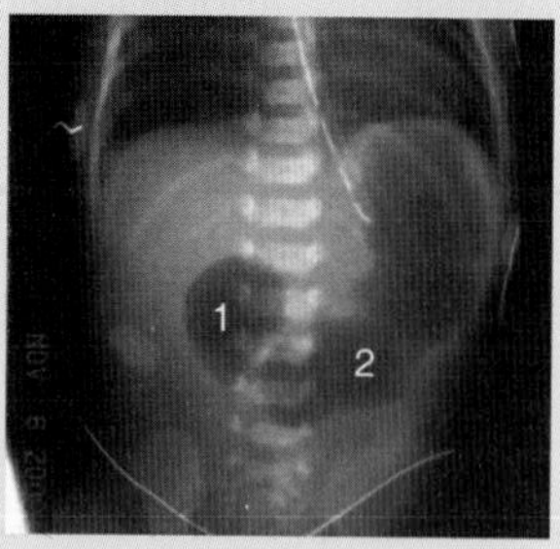 Figure 1-14. Duodenal atresia. (Reproduced with permission from Hackam DJ, et al. Pediatric surgery. In: Brunicardi F, et al., eds. *Schwartz's Principles of Surgery*. 10th ed. New York, NY: McGraw-Hill; 2014.)

The patient has warm, saline-soaked cloth placed over the gastric contents and undergoes surgery to replace the abdominal contents and close the abdominal wall defect.

Case 8: **Birth Injuries**

Setting: *Hospital*

CC: *"Why is my baby's arm not moving?"*

Vitals: *HR 150 beats/min; RR, 40 breaths/min; T: 98.6°F*

HPI: *The patient was born to a 32-year-old primipara. The pregnancy was complicated with gestational diabetes, for which the mother was taking oral hypoglycemic medications. She was often noncompliant with the medications. The mother's blood sugar seemed to be under control most of the pregnancy. The mother went into natural labor at 38 weeks' gestation and had normal labor progression. Shoulder dystocia complicated the delivery, and McRobert's maneuver was performed. The baby was delivered with the posterior shoulder first. APGAR scores at 1 and 5 minutes were 6 and 9, respectively.*

Physical Exam:
- *Head: Normal*
- *Chest: S_1S_2+ RRR no murmurs*
- *Lungs: Clear*
- *Abdomen: Normal*
- *Ext: Right arm is limp, adducted, and internally rotated. Right elbow is extended and pronated. Right wrist is flexed. Other extremities moving freely.*

Which of the following deformities is present in this patient?

a. Erb-Duchenne palsy

b. Klumpke paralysis

c. Brachial plexus paralysis

d. Spinal cord injury

e. Fracture of the humerus

Answer a. Erb-Duchenne palsy

Erb-Duchenne palsy is the "waiter's tip posture". This is adduction and internal rotation of the arm. Adduction means the arm is brought close to the body. Internal rotation means the arm is twisted in so that the palm is literally aimed behind the patient. Weakness of the biceps means the arm is extended because the biceps flexor is damaged.

Klumpke paralysis occurs when the entire hand is flaccid and there is no grip reflex present. If the entire brachial plexus were injured, then the entire arm would be flaccid, and sensory deficits would be present.

Spinal cord injuries can occur during birth, but they are most common among breech deliveries. Breech deliveries are at increased risk because the head may hyperextend during delivery. This may result in quadriplegia. If this occurs, the patients will be flaccid, but facial movements will be intact. Fractures often occur during delivery. The most commonly broken bones are the clavicles and humerus. Facial nerve palsy occurs when there are asymmetrical movements of the face. This often occurs with forceps delivery or spontaneously depending on the in utero positioning.

Which brachial roots are involved in this deformity?

a. C1 to C2

b. C2 to C3

c. C3 to C4

d. C4 to C5

e. C5 to C6

f. C6 to C7

g. C7 to C8

h. C8 to T1

Answer e. C5 to C6 (Figure 1-15)

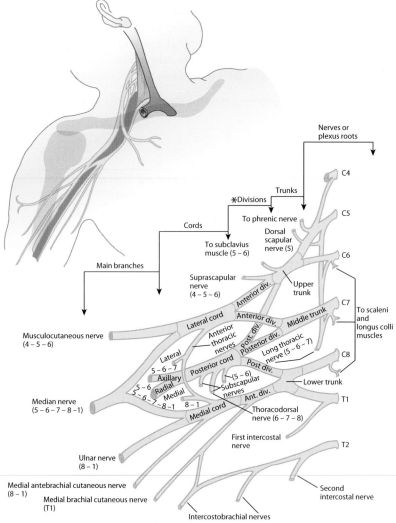

Figure 1-15. Brachial plexus. (Reproduced with permission from Waxman SG, ed. *Clinical Neuroanatomy.* 27th ed. New York, NY: McGraw-Hill; 2013.)

Erb-Duchenne palsy is associated with the nerve roots C5-C6. Klumpke Paralysis is associated with nerve roots C8-T1.

C5 Defect: Weakness of infraspinatus and deltoid muscles

C6 Defect: Biceps weakness

The patient underwent a normal nursery stay during the next 2 days. The patient is being prepared for discharge. The patient has not regained movement in his arm.

Which of the following is the next step in the management of this patient?

a. Observe the patient for 3 months

b. Physical therapy starting now

c. Surgical intervention

Answer b. Physical therapy starting now.

The patient should start physical therapy. How does a newborn do physical therapy? The parents actually do most of the work. The physical therapist will show the parents range of motion exercises and massaging that will help in the recovery of the nerve. Brachial plexus nerve palsies usually need conservative treatment because the nerve starts to regain function in a few weeks. Conservative measures in a newborn are recommended over just observation or surgical intervention.

The mother followed up with the baby's pediatrician. The infant regained movement in his arm within 4 weeks after starting physical therapy.

Case 9: Sepsis

Setting: *Office*

CC: *"My newborn has a fever."*

Vitals: *HR, 180 beats/min; RR, 60 breaths/min; T, 101.5°F*

HPI: *The patient is a 20-day-old boy who was born via NSVD at 39 weeks' gestation to a 26-year-old woman with a normal prenatal course. The mother was GBS positive at her 36th week screening and received adequate treatment during labor. The delivery and hospital stay were uneventful. The patient's APGAR score was 9 of 9. The baby has been feeding less in the past 24 hours.*

Physical Exam:

- *Gen: Awake, crying*
- *Head: NC, no cephalohematoma noted, sutures open*
- *Eyes: + Red reflex bilaterally*
- *Ears: Patent, TM normal*
- *Mouth: No cleft lip or cleft palate*
- *CVS: S_1S_2+ No murmurs heard*
- *Lungs: Clear*
- *Abd: Normal*
- *Ext: No abnormalities noted*

Which of the following is the next step in the management of this patient?

a. Refer the patient to the ED

b. Urinalysis

c. Start amoxicillin

d. Return for reevaluation tomorrow

e. No further action; reassurance that all will be well

Answer a. Refer the patient to the ED

When a patient younger than 1 month of age is found to be febrile, the patient should be sent to the ED. Febrile newborns are an emergency in pediatrics. Patients that are septic will have temperature instability. Whereas term neonates are more likely to have a fever, preterm neonates are more likely to be hypothermic.

However, if the temperature is abnormal, either up or down, in a baby, then a sepsis evaluation should be done. Sepsis evaluation should be done in the ED and includes urinalysis, blood cultures, and sometimes a lumbar puncture. Even if the urinalysis is done in the office, the patient still needs further evaluation. Do not start antibiotics before testing for the source of the infection.

On the CCS, change the location of the patient to the ED.

> *Move the clock forward 1 hour.*
>
> **Location:** *ED*
>
> *The patient's vital signs remain the same with a fever of 101.5°F.*

Which of the following is the next step in the management of this patient?

a. CBC, CMP, UA, blood cultures, urine culture

b. CBC, CMP, UA, blood cultures, urine culture, lumbar puncture

c. CBC, CMP, UA, blood cultures, urine culture, CT scan

Answer b. CBC, CMP, UA, blood cultures, urine culture, lumbar puncture

If the child is younger than 1 month of age with a documented fever, a complete sepsis workup, including lumbar puncture, should be done.

> *Move the clock forward 1 hour.*
>
> • *CBC: WBC count is 15,000; platelet count is 350,000*
> • *CMP: within normal limits*
> • *UA: Negative*

Mechanism of leukocytosis in fever
• 50% of WBCs are on "margins" or walls of blood vessels.
• Epinephrine and glucocorticoids go up in febrile stress.
• Epinephrine and glucocorticoids signal the WBCs to come off the walls.
• Expect a doubling of WBC count in all severe stress.

What is the next step in the management of this baby?

a. Start ampicillin

b. Start ampicillin and gentamicin

c. Start ampicillin, gentamicin, and ceftriaxone

d. Wait for the results of cultures

e. Infectious diseases consultation

Answer b. Start ampicillin and gentamicin.

Newborns with a fever and elevated WBC count are likely to be septic. Empiric treatment for sepsis is ampicillin and gentamicin. The most common pathogens responsible for sepsis in the newborn are GBS and *Escherichia coli*. Ceftriaxone is contraindicated in newborns because it is highly protein bound and could displace bilirubin, leading to jaundice and kernicterus. In infants younger than 30 days of age, ceftriaxone should be avoided.

The whole point of the question is that you cannot wait for the result of culture in a febrile, ill neonate. You do not need an infectious disease consultant to do these tests and order basic antibiotics such as ampicillin and gentamicin.

Mechanism of ceftriaxone excretion
- Ceftriaxone is excreted by glucuronidation in the bile.
- The enzymatic machinery for glucuronidation is not fully functional in newborns.

After 36 hours of antibiotics, all culture results are negative. The baby is discharged home without complications.

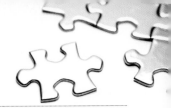

CHAPTER 2

GENETICS

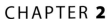

CASE 1: Abnormal Number of Chromosomes

Setting: *Office*

CC: *"My child is not meeting his milestones."*

Vitals: *HR, 110 beats/min; RR, 30 breaths/min*

HPI: *A 1-year-old boy is brought to the office because his mother states that he is not meeting developmental milestones. The mother states that the patient did not start to sit alone 10 or 11 months of age and still is not walking. The patient is not even crawling yet.*

Physical Exam: *Generalized hypotonia (Figure 2-1)*

Which chromosomal abnormality does this patient have?

a. Trisomy 13

b. Trisomy 18

c. Trisomy 21

d. Turner syndrome

e. Klinefelter syndrome

Answer c. Trisomy 21

See the table below for a description of the most tested genetic syndromes.

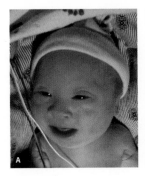
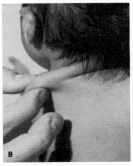
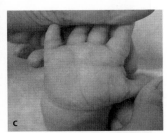

Figure 2-1. (A) Down syndrome facies (B) Nuchal skin (C) Simian crease. (Reproduced with permission from Cunningham F, et al. Genetics. In: Cunningham F, et al., eds. *Williams Obstetrics.* 24th ed. New York, NY: McGraw-Hill; 2013.)

Chromosomal Disorders

Disease	Type of Chromosomal Disorder	Physical Exam Findings	Associated Disorders
Down syndrome	Trisomy 21	• Upslanting palpebral fissures • Epicanthal folds • Midface hypoplasia • Generalized hypotonia	• Endocardial cushion defects • Duodenal atresia • Acute lymphoblastic leukemia
Edwards syndrome	Trisomy 18	• Growth retardation • Hypertonicity • Rocker-bottom feet • Overlapping fingers	• Heart failure and pneumonia usually cause death in infancy
Patau syndrome	Trisomy 13	• Eye malformations • Cleft lip and palate • Polydactyly	• Usually incompatible with life
Turner syndrome	XO	• Webbed neck • Triangular face • Short stature • Wide-set nipples • Amenorrhea • Edema in extremities	• Coarctation of the aorta • Normal IQ • Learning disabilities

Klinefelter syndrome	XXY	• Microorchidism • Lack of libido • Tall, eunuchoid body • Gynecomastia	• Usually found during infertility work up • Azoospermia • Sterility
Neurofibromatosis type I	Autosomal dominant	• Café- au-lait spot • Neurofibromas	
Cystic fibrosis	Autosomal recessive	• *CFTR* gene alteration • Abnormal exchange at the NaCl receptor	• Buildup of thick mucus in lungs, digestive tract, and pancreas
Prader-Willi syndrome	15q11-13 from paternal inheritance (genomic imprinting)	• Hyperphagia leading to obesity • Hypotonia (from birth) • Cognitive impairment	• Type II DM • Sleep apnea • Diseases associated with obesity
Angelman syndrome	15q11-13 from maternal inheritance (genomic imprinting)	• "Happy puppet" • Severe intellectual impairment • Frequent laughter • Excitable personality	• Seizures

Neurofibromas are benign tumors consisting of Schwann cells, nerve fibers, and fibroblasts.

Neurofibromatosis type I has neurofibromas all over the body.

Neurofibromatosis type II is associated with bilateral acoustic neuromas and minimal skin lesions.

Autosomal dominant disorders
• Neurofibromatosis
• Marfan syndrome
• Osteogenesis imperfecta

Autosomal recessive disorders
• Cystic fibrosis
• Inborn errors of metabolism
• Tay-Sachs disease

Sex chromosome disorders
• Turner syndrome
• Klinefelter syndrome
• XYY and XXX

Genomic imprinting
• Different diseases depending on the parent that the gene was inherited from
    • Angelman syndrome = MATERNAL
    • Prader-Willi syndrome = PATERNAL

How was this genetic disorder inherited?

a. Nondisjunction during mitosis   **c.** Mendelian genetics
b. Nondisjunction during meiosis   **d.** Multifactorial inheritance

Answer a. Nondisjunction during meiosis

Trisomy 21 and all trisomy disorders are the failure of the chromosomes to separate during meiosis. Mitosis creates two new daughter cells, and meiosis creates four daughter cells.

One of the daughter cells will have two chromosome 21s, and one of the daughter cells will have no chromosome 21s Mendelian genetics includes the autosomal dominant and recessive disorders. Multifactorial inheritance does not have one clear inheritance pathway but a combination of the genes working together (Figure 2-2).

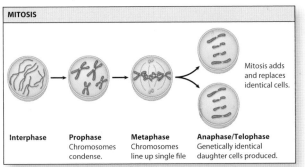

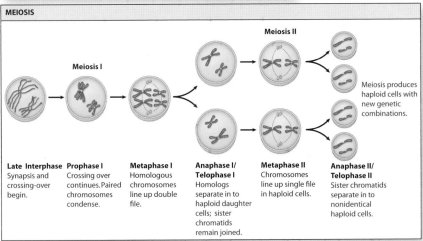

Figure 2-2. (Reproduced with permission from Mescher AL. Chapter 3. The nucleus. In: Mescher AL, eds. *Junqueira's Basic Histology: Text & Atlas.* 13th ed. New York, NY: McGraw-Hill; 2013.)

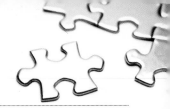

CHAPTER **3**

GROWTH AND DEVELOPMENT

CASE 1: Milestones

Setting: *Office*

CC: *"Is my child developing normally?"*

Vitals: *HR, 120 beats/min, RR, 25 breaths/min*

HPI: *A 2-month-old girl is brought to the office for her well-child checkup. The patient is currently smiling, has good head control, and is cooing. The patient turns her head towards sounds and follows things with her eyes. During tummy time, the patient holds her head up but does not seem to respond to loud noises.*

Physical Exam:
- *Gen: Awake, crying*
- *Head: Normocephalic, no cephalohematoma noted, sutures open*
- *Eyes: Red reflex is present bilaterally*
- *Ears: Tympanic membranes normal*
- *Mouth: No cleft lip or cleft palate*
- *CVS: Normal*
- *Lungs: Clear*
- *Abd: Normal*
- *Ext: No abnormalities noted, negative Barlow and Ortolani*

Which of the following qualities could be a possible developmental delay?

a. Smiles

b. Turns head toward sound

c. Follows things with her eyes

d. Does not respond to loud noises

e. Holds up head

Answer d. Does not respond to loud noises

These are the 2-month-old milestones. Milestones are broken down into physical development, cognitive development, communication development, and social development.

Children develop at different ranges; there is a range of what is considered normal. If the patient does not start responding to loud sounds by the next visit, a full workup should be done, including a hearing test.

Below, find a chart of the developmental milestones that should be assessed:

Developmental Milestones

Age	Social	Language	Cognitive	Physical
2 months	• Smiles at people • Tries to look at parents	• Coos • Turns head to sounds	• Follows things with eyes • Is fussy if activity is not stimulating	• Holds head up during tummy time • Makes smoother movements with extremities
4 months	• Copies facial expressions	• Babbles • Copies sounds • Cries in different ways to convey message	• Responds to affection • Reaches for objects • Follows moving objects • Recognizes familiar faces	• Rolls from tummy to back • Holds toy and shakes it • Puts hands to mouth • Can push up to elbows
6 months	• Plays with parents • Looks at self in mirror	• Babbles vowels • Responds to his or her name • Can show joy and displeasure	• Puts objects to his or her mouth • Passes things from hand to hand	• Rolls over both directions • Sits without support
9 months	• Shows stranger anxiety • Clings to familiar adults	• Understands NO • Copies gestures • Can point with fingers	• Plays peek-a-boo • Looks for things when they fall • Uses pincher grasp	• Stands while holding on • Pulls to stand • Crawls
1 year	• Cries when parents leave • Has favorite things • Has fear • Puts arm or leg out to aid in dressing	• Responds correctly to directions • Waves and shakes head no • Says "mama" and "dada"	• Bangs things together • Points with index finger • Puts things in a container	• Stands alone • Cruises (walks along the furniture) • Takes a few steps alone

Age				
18 months	• Hands things to others • Plays simple pretend • Explores with parents	• Says single-word sentences • Says "yes" and "no"	• Points to body parts • Follows one-step verbal commands • Scribbles	• Walks alone • Walk up steps • Drinks from cup
2 years	• Independent • Plays beside other children • Exhibits defiant behavior	• Points to things or pictures when named • Says two- to four-word sentences • Repeats words heard in conversations	• Sorts shapes and colors • Completes sentences • Makes believe • Builds a tower of four or more blocks	• Kicks ball • Runs • Goes up and down stairs • Throws ball overhand
3 years	• Copies adults • Shows affection • Takes turns in games • Gets upset with major changes in routine	• Follows two- or three-step commands • Names friends • Says first name, age, and sex • Says two- or three-word sentences	• Makes believe with dolls or animals • Copies a circle when drawing • Turns a book pages one at a time • Builds a tower of six or more blocks	• Climbs well • Rides a tricycle • Goes up and down stairs alternating feet
4 years	• Likes new things • Wants to play with others • Is more creative • Talks about likes	• Uses basic grammar • Tells stories • Sing songs • Knows first and last name	• Knows colors and numbers • Uses scissors • Draws a person with two to four body parts	• Stands on one foot • Pours or cuts own food • Catches a bouncing ball
5 years	• Wants to be like friends • Agrees to rules • Is gender aware	• Tells a whole story • Uses future tense • Knows name and address	• Can draw a person with six body parts • Copies triangle • Can write some letters and numbers	• Hops and skips • Somersaults • Swings and climbs • Is potty trained

CASE 2: Immunizations

Setting: *Office*

CC: *"Which immunizations does my child need?"*

Vitals: *HR, 110 beats/min; RR, 25 breaths/min*

HPI: *A 2-month-old boy presents with his mother for his well-child visit. The mother had routine prenatal care and an uneventful delivery. The baby has gained 2 pounds in the past month and grown 1 inch. The baby is smiling often, cooing, and trying to hold his head up. He is eating every 3 or 4 hours.*

Which of the following vaccinations or combination of vaccinations should be given?

a. Hepatitis A, Hib, and polio

b. MMR, DTap, and polio

c. DTap, polio, pneumococcal, rotavirus, and Hib

d. Varicella, MMR, and DTap

e. Hepatitis B and hepatitis A and Hib

Answer c. DTap, polio, pneumococcal, rotavirus, and Hib

Patients who are 2 months old should receive DTap (diphtheria, tetanus, and pertussis), polio, pneumococcal, Hib (*Haemophilus influenzae* type b), and rotavirus vaccinations. These vaccinations will be repeated at 2, 4, and 6 months of age.

Rotavirus vaccine is given at 2, 4, and 6 months old. After 6 months old, this vaccination is no longer given. It is not including in the catch-up vaccinations unless the child is younger than 6 months old.

Hepatitis A, MMR (measles, mumps, and rubella), and varicella vaccinations are given at 1 year of age.

Hepatitis B vaccinations are given at birth, 1 to 2 months, and again at 6 months to 1 year old.

See the vaccination schedule according to the Centers for Disease Control and Prevention in Figure 3-1.

The way this chart is read is to start with the age of the patient. Let's take an example. If the child is 12 months old, then the patient should have had the third hepatitis B vaccination (may receive it from 6 months to 18 months old), fourth pneumococcal vaccination (may receive from 12–15 months) third polio vaccination (6–18 months), MMR vaccination (12–15 months), varicella vaccination (12–15 months), and hepatitis A vaccination (12–23 months). Then ensure the patient has had all of these vaccinations by the end of the graphed time slot.

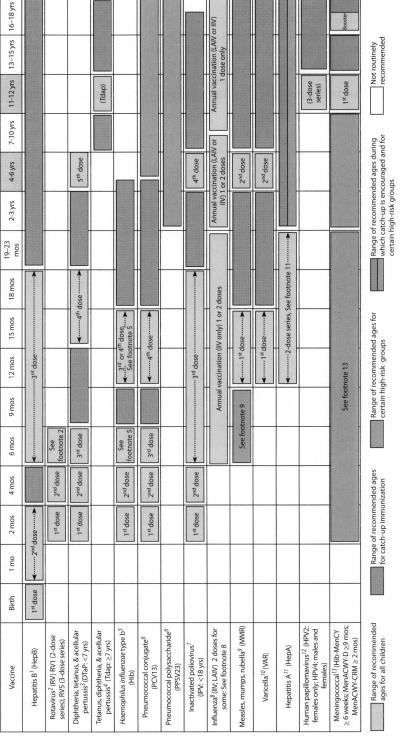

Figure 3-1. Childhood Immunization Schedule. (Reprinted from CDC.gov. http://www.cdc.gov/vaccines/schedules/downloads/child/0-18yrs-schedule.pdf.)

> *The proper vaccines are given to the patient, and he develops a fever of 100.7°F that night. His mother calls the office upset because the vaccinations made her child sick.*

Which of the following is the next step in the management of this patient?

a. Come to the office for evaluation

b. Take ibuprofen

c. Take acetaminophen

d. Take amoxicillin

Answer c. Take acetaminophen.

Fever after administration of vaccines is a common side effect, one that should be explained to parents before administration. The body is fighting the vaccine to build antibodies.

Ibuprofen should not given to children unless they are 6 months of age or older. Acetaminophen is the treatment of choice for a 2-month-old infant with a fever from vaccinations. If the fever persists for more than 1 to 2 days or the child is exhibiting other signs of illness, then the patient should be brought in for evaluation. Never treat patients with antibiotics without examining them first.

Rotavirus = Reoviridae
• Causes severe diarrhea
Contraindications to vaccinations
• Moderate to severe acute illness
• No live virus in if not immunocompetent

> *The mother states that after taking the acetaminophen, the child has improved rapidly. In 24 hours, the fever is gone.*

CASE 3: Enuresis

Setting: *Office*

CC: *"My child is wetting the bed."*

Vitals: *HR, 90 beats/min; RR, 25 breaths/min*

HPI: *A 5-year-old boy with no past medical history is brought to the office by his mother for frequent nighttime bed wetting. The mother states that he was previously sleeping through the night without wetting his bed for about 6 or 7 months. But for the last several weeks, he has been wetting the bed every night. The patient's mother states that there has been a recent change of a new sibling in the home. The patient is continent during the day and does not seem to hold his urine excessively.*

Which of the following is the most likely diagnosis at this time?

a. Primary enuresis

b. Secondary enuresis

c. Bladder dysfunction

d. Urinary tract infection (UTI)

Answer b. Secondary enuresis

The bladder becomes mature at 5 years old. Before age 5 years, it is unrealistic that children will be able to hold urine for prolonged periods of time. Primary enuresis is most common and means that a child has never had a dry period. Secondary enuresis is followed by a period of at least 6 months of dryness. Secondary enuresis is often manifested when the child becomes stressed, such as with the birth of a new sibling. Bladder dysfunction occurs when the patient not only has nocturnal symptoms but daytime symptoms as well. This can be related to UTI, detrusor instability, or neurologic disorders.

Which of the following is the next step in the management of this patient?

a. Urinalysis

b. Renal ultrasonography

c. Postvoid residual volume

d. Abdominal radiography

Answer a. Urinalysis

A urinalysis is always the first step in assessing enuresis. Enuresis may be the first sign of a UTI. Renal ultrasonography, postvoid residual, and abdominal radiography may be done as part of a workup of enuresis. However, these tests are usually reserved for primary enuresis or patients with daytime symptoms.

After a few weeks of adjustment, the child still continues to wet the bed at night.

Which of the following measures is most effective?

a. Drinking less water through out the day

b. Using a nighttime alarm

c. Yelling at the child when he wets the bed

d. Making the child clean up the bed

e. Psychotherapy

Answer b. Using a nighttime alarm

Both yelling at the child and making him clean up the bed are negative feedback for the child. These methods are not effective and just make the child's self-confidence decrease. Drinking less water throughout the day is not necessary, but restricting drinks before bed is helpful. The most effective way to help the child is to set a nighttime alarm. If a parent wakes the child during the night to use the bathroom, it will be less likely that the child will wet the bed. However, the parents are inconvenienced by this method and often have resistance to it.

> After several weeks of nighttime alarms, the child continues to have enuresis. The tests results are within normal limits.

Which of the following is the next best step in the management of this patient?

a. Continue nighttime alarms

b. No further management is needed

c. Desmopressin

d. Amitriptyline

Answer c. Desmopressin

Desmopressin is the first-line treatment in children with nocturnal enuresis that has failed conservative management such as decreased fluid intake before bed and nighttime alarms. If the patient has failed nighttime alarms, alternate treatment should be sought. Amitriptyline and imipramine are tricyclic antidepressants (TCAs) that are used in enuresis that is refractory to desmopressin. They are less efficacious and have more adverse effects than desmopressin.

> After administration of desmopressin, the child improves, and no further management is needed.

Mechanism of desmopressin
- Desmopressin is antidiuretic hormone
- Increases water reabsorption at collecting duct
- Stimulates V2 receptors
- Inserts aquaporins at the collecting duct
- Decreases urine volume

Mechanism of the TCAs
- Acetylcholine leads to bladder constriction.
- TCAs are anticholinergic.
- TCAs inhibit detrusor muscle activity.
- TCAs decrease both the frequency and force of bladder contractions.

CASE 4: Encopresis

Setting: *Office*

CC: *"My child has fecal incontinence."*

Vitals: *HR, 90 beats/min; RR, 20 breaths/min*

HPI: *The patient is a 5-year-old boy with no past medical history who is brought to the office by his mother for fecal incontinence. The mother states that the boy is very embarrassed but soils himself more than two times a week.*

Physical Exam: *Within normal limits, including rectal exam and rectal tone*

Which of the following is the most common cause of encopresis?

a. Sexual abuse

b. Anatomic disturbances

c. Constipation

d. Hypotonia

Answer c. Constipation

The most common reason for fecal incontinence is constipation. Knowing the stool consistency, volume, and frequency is imperative to making the diagnosis. Some children may have daily bowel movements but fail to completely evacuate the bowel. The other choices are all reasons for constipation, but the most common cause is constipation.

CASE 5: Autism

Setting: *Office*

CC: *"My son is not speaking."*

HPI: *An 18-month-old boy presents to the office with his mother for concerns about his speech. The mother states that he used to speak five or six words. The mother states that the patient seems to have forgotten how to speak. The patient is walking alone, trying to climb the stairs, and likes to scribble on paper.*

Physical Exam: *Within normal limits; minimal interaction with physician or parents*

Which of the following is the next step in the management of this patient?

a. Assure the mother that this is normal

b. Refer to early intervention

c. Computed tomography (CT) of the head

d. Hearing test

Answer d. Hearing test

Any time there is a concern about the patient's language development, a hearing test should be done. At 18 months, the patient should be able to speak one-word sentences and respond yes and no, and he should be building his vocabulary. The most common reason for language delay is a hearing problem. Before the patient is referred to early intervention, a hearing issue should be ruled out. It is hard for a child to interact with others when he cannot hear them. CT of the head is not done as a first test in developmental delay.

The patient is sent for an audiology evaluation; results are normal.

Which of the following is the next step in the management of this patient?

a. Send patient for otolaryngology evaluation

b. Send patient to early intervention

c. Ages and Stages Questionnaire (ASQ)

d. Send patient to genetics

Answer b. Early intervention

The patient is experiencing some red flags for autism, including language delay and social interaction issues. Any patient who is thought to possibly have autism should be sent directly to early intervention or neurodevelopmental for evaluations. ENT or otolaryngology evaluation and genetics are not valid referrals in autism. The ASQ is a parental question-naire that is done as a part of the routine check-up at 9 months, 1 year, and 18 months.

Vaccines are not a cause of autism.

There is a spectrum of autism, ranging from mild to severe.
• Must have two components: problems with social communication and interaction and repetitive patterns
• Restricted and repetitive behaviors

The patient is sent to early intervention and was diagnosed is Asperger syndrome.

DSM-5 Criteria for Autism versus Asperger Syndrome

Autism	Asperger Syndrome
A: Impairment in social interaction	A: Impairment in social interaction
1. Marked impairment of nonverbal behaviors (eye-to-eye contact)	5. Marked impairment of nonverbal behaviors (eye-to-eye contact)
2. No peer relationships	6. No peer relationships
3. Lack of spontaneous seeking to share enjoyment	7. Lack of spontaneous seeking to share enjoyment
4. Lack of emotional reciprocity	8. Lack of emotional reciprocity
(Must have two of these items)	(Must have two of these items)
B: Impairment in communication	B: Repetitive and stereotyped behavior
1. Delay or lack of development of spoken language	5. Preoccupation with stereotyped and restricted patterns of interest
2. In patients with speech, marked impairment in the ability to initiate or sustain conversation with others	6. Inflexible adherence to specific routines
	7. Repetitive motor mannerisms
3. Repetitive use of language	8. Preoccupation with parts of objects
4. Lack of make-believe play	(Must have one of these items)
(Must have one of these items)	

Autism	Asperger Syndrome
C: Repetitive and stereotyped behavior 1. Preoccupation with stereotyped and restricted patterns of interest 2. Inflexible adherence to specific routines 3. Repetitive motor mannerisms 4. Preoccupation with parts of objects (Must have one of these items) Patient must have a total of six from all three categories.	
Delays in the following areas, with the onset before 3 years old: • Social interaction • Language use at social interaction • Symbolic or imaginative play	Clinically significant impairments in social and occupational functioning
	No delay in language
	No delay in cognitive development or in the development of age-appropriate self-help skills or adaptive behaviors
	Criteria for other pervasive and developmental disorders and schizophrenia not met

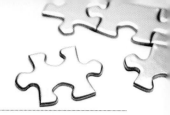

CHAPTER **4**

RESPIRATORY DISEASES

CASE 1: Bronchiolitis

Setting: *Office*

CC: *"My 6-month-old can't breathe."*

HPI: *A 6-month-old baby with no prenatal history and a negative past medical history presents to the office for shortness of breath and a cough. The mother states that since the winter started, the child has been coughing more frequently. However, in the past 2 days, he has been unable to stop coughing and seems to be short of breath. The patient does attend daycare.*

ROS:
- *Shortness of breath present*
- *Negative for fever, chills*
- *Positive for decreased appetite*
- *Posttussive vomiting is present*

Physical Exam:
- *Baby is awake and alert, lying on back with intercostal retractions*
- *Wheezing diffusely*
- *Heart is normal*
- *Ears, nose, and throat are normal*

Which of the following is the next step in the management of this patient?

a. Chest radiography (CXR)

b. Albuterol

c. Surfactant

d. Prednisone

Answer b. Albuterol

In the outpatient setting, the next step in the management of a baby with respiratory distress and wheezing is to obtain pulse oximetry, usually on a finger or toe, and start to administer albuterol.

Which class of drug is albuterol?

a. β_2-Adrenergic agonist

b. Anticholinergic

c. Corticosteroid

d. α_1-Adrenergic agonist

Answer a. β_2-Adrenergic agonist

Albuterol is a short-acting β_2-adrenergic agonist. α_1-Adrenergic agonists stimulate phospholipase C activity, causing vasoconstriction and mydriasis. An example is midodrine (used to increase blood pressure). Anticholinergic drugs are broken down into antimuscarinic agents and antinicotinic agents. An example of antimuscarinic anticholinergic medication used in asthma and chronic obstructive pulmonary disease is tiotropium (Spiriva). Corticosteroids mimic steroid hormones, and they may be administered systemically or inhaled.

> *The patient's pulse oximeter shows 89% saturation before the administration of albuterol. After the administration of albuterol, the patient's pulse oximetry increases to 95%.*

Which of the following is the most likely diagnosis?

a. Pneumonia

b. Bronchitis

c. Bronchiolitis

d. Cystic fibrosis (CF)

Answer c. Bronchiolitis

Bronchiolitis is inflammation of the smallest airways. It is the most common form of respiratory problems in children age 3 to 6 months old, but it may occur up until 2 years of age (Figure 4-1). Bronchiolitis most commonly presents with shortness of breath, wheezing, and cough. Other symptoms include poor feeding, apnea, nasal flaring, intercostal retractions, and lethargy. Bronchitis is inflammation in the medium to large airways, leading to cough and coarse breath sounds. It often occurs in older children and adults.

Pneumonia occurs when a collection of inflammation and infection occurs in specific location in the lungs. CF is an autosomal recessive condition leading to thick mucus. The child will have poor growth and malnutrition despite normal food intake. Patients are also at increased risk for multiple lung infections. This child currently has an acute infection; CF may be underlying, but it would be too soon to tell.

> *The patient is sent home on albuterol nebulizers. The mother is told to bring the child back to the office in 2 or 3 days.*

Which of the following is the most common cause of bronchiolitis in this population?

a. Influenza

b. Strep pneumonia

c. Respiratory syncytial virus (RSV)

d. *Haemophilus influenzae* type B (Hib)

e. Bordetella pertussis

Answer c. Respiratory syncytial virus (RSV)

The most common cause of bronchiolitis in children is RSV. Strep pneumonia is the most common cause of pneumonia. Influenza can cause wheezing, but it is not the most common cause of bronchiolitis. Hib causes epiglottitis. Bordetella pertussis is the cause of whooping cough.

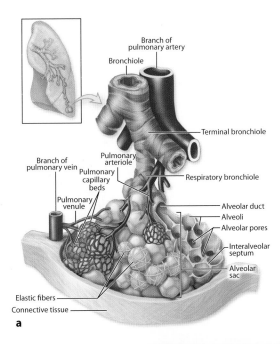

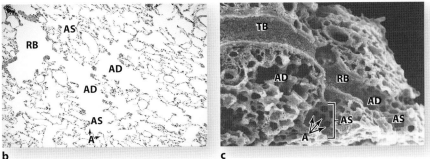

Figure 4-1. Anatomy of respiratory tree. (Reproduced with permission from Mescher AL. Chapter 17. The respiratory system. In: Mescher AL, eds. *Junqueira's Basic Histology: Text & Atlas*. 13th ed. New York, NY: McGraw-Hill; 2013.)

RSV
• Single-stranded RNA virus
• Paramyxoviridae

Influenza
• Single-stranded RNA virus
• Orthomyxoviridae

Strep pneumonia (Figure 4-2)
• Gram-positive, α-hemolytic bacteria

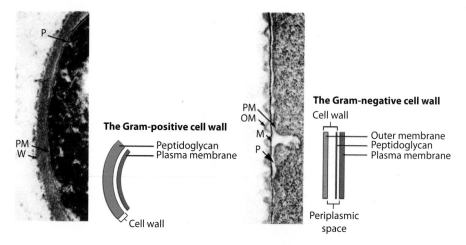

Figure 4-2. Gram positive vs gram negative. (Reproduced with permission from Ryan KJ, Ray C. Bacteria—basic concepts. In: Ryan KJ, Ray C, eds. *Sherris Medical Microbiology*. 6th ed. New York, NY: McGraw-Hill; 2014. Fig. 21-4.)

Hib
- Gram-negative coccobacilli
- Pasteurellaceae

Bordetella pertussis
- Gram-negative coccobacilli
- Proteobacteria

The patient returns to the office several days later. He is improved and is no longer using the nebulizer.

Which of the following risk factors would put that child at risk for a poor outcome?

a. Healthy baby

b. Born at 39 weeks' gestation

c. Patient with CF

Answer c. Patient with CF

Patients with underlying cardiac or pulmonary disease are at risk for increased mortality from RSV. Risk factors for poor outcomes with RSV bronchiolitis are prematurity, severe illness, cardiac disease, and pulmonary disease.

How could this be prevented in this patient?

a. Hand washing

b. Vaccination against RSV

c. Palivizumab

d. N-Acetylcysteine

Answer a. Hand washing

The child in the question is a healthy baby who was born full term. Currently, because the disease in healthy children is usually self-limited, the only way to prevent the infection is by hand washing. There is no vaccine for RSV. Palivizumab is a humanized monoclonal antibody against RSV glycoproteins. It is only indicated in premature children, children with congenital heart disease, and children with bronchopulmonary disease.

CASE 2: Acute Asthma Exacerbation

Setting: *Office*

CC: *"My child has a cough."*

HPI: *A 5-year-old boy is brought to the office by his mother for cough and shortness of breath. He has been coughing, wheezing, and short of breath for 2 days. The mother states that he has also had a fever of 101.2°F and a runny nose.*

Physical Exam:
- *Nasal congestion present*
- *Mild tonsillar erythema*
- *Wheezing in bilateral lungs*
- *Intercostal retraction*
- *Unable to complete full sentences*
- *Pulse oximetry: 83% on room air*

Which of the following is the next step in the management of this patient?

a. Administer albuterol

b. Transfer to the emergency department (ED)

c. Administer racemic epinephrine

d. Administer theophylline

e. Administer inhaled steroids

Answer a. Administer albuterol

This patient is wheezing, tipping us off to a probable asthma attack. Asthma exacerbations are often precipitated by viral infections, as indicated by the runny nose and fever. Albuterol should be used as the first method of increasing the pulse oximetry measurement. Opening up the bronchioles this will allow the patient to breathe more oxygen.

Transfer to the ED may be necessary, but start therapy first! Albuterol opens up the airways of the lungs. Racemic epinephrine is used in whooping cough.

Theophylline is never an acute rescue medication. Theophylline is occasionally used as chronic therapy when β-agonists, inhaled steroids, and leukotriene antagonists are not effective. Inhaled steroids are great long-term controller medications but are never used as an acute rescue medication.

Which of the following is the next step in the management of this patient?

a. Administer oxygen

b. Administer albuterol

c. Give magnesium

d. Administer terbutaline

e. Administer isoproterenol

Answer b. Administer albuterol

The patient's pulse oxygen is still low; it is improving but is still low. Administer more albuterol and consider transferring the patient to the ED. Oxygen is not going open up the lungs. Magnesium is not given in a pediatrician's office because toxicity can lead to severe hypotension, arrhythmias, and cardiac arrest.

Isoproterenol is a nonspecific β-agonist with no clinical utility. Isoproterenol has not been used as a clinical medication for more than 30 years. Neither terbutaline nor isoproterenol has greater clinical efficacy than albuterol.

> *The patient's pulse oxygen is increased to 87% with one dose of albuterol. He continues to be wheezing bilaterally and have intercostal retractions. He is transferred to the ED. In the ED, the patient is found to be dyspneic and wheezing. The patient continues to have shortness of breath, cough, and wheezing. His pulse oxygen is 87%.*

Magnesium relaxes muscle!
- Magnesium is useful as a tocolytic agent because it relaxes the muscle of the uterus.
- Magnesium relaxes smooth muscle surrounding bronchi.

Which of the following is the next step in the management of this patient?

a. Administer methylprednisolone

b. CXR

c. Arterial blood gas (ABG) analysis

d. Intubate the child

Answer a. Administer methylprednisolone

The child is still in respiratory distress; at this point, multiple things will be occurring at the same time. A CXR and ABG analysis will be done, but they will only provide information on why this may be occurring. These tests will not make the child breathe better. Methylprednisolone is a glucocorticoid that should be given to help reduce the inflammation in the airways. The child will also be receiving albuterol, ipratropium, and oxygen. This will help the child breathe better. Intubation will start to be considered but is always the last treatment option.

> *After administration of steroids, albuterol, and ipratropium, the patient's pulse ox increases to 95%. Upon discharge, the patient will be given albuterol and decreasing doses of steroids.*

Mechanism of ipratropium
• Inhibitor of acetylcholine
• Dilates bronchi
• Ipratropium and tiotropium decrease mucous gland output
• Nonabsorbed quaternary amines
• Similar to nonabsorbed atropine

CASE 3: Asthma

Setting: *Office*

CC: *"My child coughs a lot at night."*

Vitals: *T, 98.5°F; HR, 90 beats/min; RR, 20 breaths/min; pulse ox, 99%*

HPI: *A 7-year-old girl is brought to the office by her mother, who states that the child seems to always be coughing at night. The mother states that the patient often awakens in the middle of the night coughing and gasping for breath. The patient has not been given any medications previously. The patient states that she sometimes has to stop playing at school because of the cough.*

Physical Exam:
- *Awake, alert, oriented*
- *Tympanic membranes are normal bilaterally*
- *Pharynx is normal*
- *Lungs are clear to auscultation bilaterally*
- *Heart sounds are normal*

Which of the following is the most likely diagnosis for this patient?

a. Allergic rhinitis
b. Aspiration
c. Bronchiectasis
d. Cough-variant asthma
e. Pertussis

Answer d. Cough-variant asthma

The most common diagnosis is cough-variant asthma. The tip-off that this is cough-variant asthma is that the patient is healthy otherwise with no physical examination findings. Allergic rhinitis would occur during specific times of the year or when in contact with the allergen. On physical examination, the nasal turbinates would be enlarged, and a cobblestone pattern would be present in the pharynx. Although this is not always true in life, on the boards, if they want you to know the answer, they have to tell you something! Aspiration would generally occur in a newborn who is choking with feedings. Bronchiectasis would have hemoptysis or a wet cough. Pertussis would have the classic seal-like cough. Pertussis is an infection, so it would happen throughout the day, not only at specific times (i.e., during activity or at night).

Which of the following is the treatment of choice for this patient?

a. Short-acting β-agonist
b. Long-acting β-agonist
c. Low-dose inhaled glucocorticoids
d. High-dose inhaled glucocorticoids

Answer a. Short-acting β-agonist

All of the treatments above are used in asthma, but they are used in a stepwise fashion. As the asthma worsens, the more medications are used.

Cough-variant asthma should be treated with a short-acting β-agonist, such as albuterol. Albuterol is used as a rescue treatment during acute exacerbations as well as in the milder cases of asthma.

After several years of the child being stable on the initial treatment, she presents to the office with worsening symptoms. The patient, now 12 years old, states that she is now feeling shortness of breath and is using her inhaler three or four times a week. She also states that she wakes up at night to use the inhaler once a week.

Physical Exam:
- *Within normal limits*

Which of the following is the classification of the patient's asthma?

a. Cough variant

b. Intermittent

c. Mild persistent

d. Moderate persistent

e. Severe persistent

Answer c. Mild persistent

Asthma classification is based on a collection of symptoms and the frequency of the symptoms. They are split into the following categories: symptoms, nighttime awakenings, the need for the rescue inhaler, interference with normal activity, and spirometer results.

Classification of Asthma

Severity	Symptom Frequency	Nighttime Symptoms	% FEV$_1$ of Predicted	FEV$_1$ Variability	Short-Acting β-Agonist
Intermittent	<2/week	<2/month	>80%	20%	<2/day
Mild persistent	>2/week	3–4/month	>80%	20%–30%	>2/day
Moderate persistent	Daily	>1/week	60%–80%	>30%	Daily
Severe persistent	Continuous	Frequent	<60%	>30%	>2/day

FEV$_1$, forced expiratory volume in 1 second.

The patient is correctly diagnosed.

Which of the following is the treatment of choice?

a. Albuterol only

b. Albuterol and low-dose inhaled corticosteroid

c. Albuterol and medium-dose inhaled corticosteroid

d. Long-acting β-agonist and high-dose inhaled corticosteroids

e. Oral steroids

Answer b. Albuterol and low-dose inhaled corticosteroid

Mild persistent asthma treatment starts with low-dose inhaled corticosteroids and albuterol. As the symptoms worsen, a new drug is added to the treatment. Moderate persistent asthma is treated with albuterol and medium-dose inhaled corticosteroids. Severe persistent asthma is treated with long-acting β-agonists and high-dose inhaled corticosteroids.

CASE 4: Pneumonia

Setting: *Office*

CC: *"My child has a cough and fever."*

Vitals: *T, 101.1°F; HR, 96 beats/min; RR, 21 breath/min; pulse ox, 94%*

HPI: *A 7-year-old girl with no past medical history presents to the office with her mother for 1 week of cough and fever. The mother states that the child has been coughing up greenish-looking sputum. She also has a runny nose, temperature of 101.1°F, and posttussive vomiting.*

Physical Exam:
- *Lung exam is positive for crackles in left lower lung field*
- *Otherwise within normal limits*

Types of Pneumonia

Type of Pneumonia	Question Hint	Treatment
Community-acquired pneumonia	Normal healthy child	Amoxicillin or azithromycin
Hospital-acquired pneumonia	In the hospital in the past 30 days	Two-drug regimen: aminoglycoside (gentamicin) and gram-positive anaerobe killer (meropenem, piperacillin–tazobactam, or ceftazidime)
Aspiration pneumonia	Episode of choking	Amoxicillin–clavulanate or clindamycin

Which type of pneumonia does this patient most likely have?

a. Community acquired
b. Nosocomial
c. Aspiration

Answer a. Community acquired pneumonia

Which of the following is the next step in the management of this patient?

a. Azithromycin
b. Doxycycline
c. Ciprofloxacin
d. Clindamycin
e. Oseltamivir

Answer a. Azithromycin

Azithromycin and the macrolides are the initial drugs of choice in children older than 5 years of age with community-acquired pneumonia. Doxycycline is not given to children younger than 8 years of age. Ciprofloxacin is not used in the treatment of pneumonia. Clindamycin is used in aspiration pneumonia. Oseltamivir is used in pneumonia secondary to the flu.

The patient is given the proper antibiotic but returns 2 days later. The patient is complaining of worsening cough, shortness of breath, and decreased appetite.

Vitals: *T, 100.9°F; HR, 101 beats/min; RR, 28 breaths/min; pulse ox, 89%*

ROS: *Continues to have fever and chills*

Physical Exam:
• *Patient is short of breath with intercostal retractions and crackles bilaterally*

Which of the following is the next step in the management of this patient?

a. Change to levofloxacin

b. Change to amoxicillin–clavulanate

c. Send the patient to the ED

d. Refer to pulmonology

Answer c. Send the patient to the ED

The patient has gotten worse while taking antibiotics. There are now two reasons to send the patient to the ED: She failed outpatient treatment and is not breathing well.

Indications for inpatient treatment
• Hypoxia (pulse oximetry <90%)
• Dehydration or unable to tolerate oral intake
• Severe respiratory distress (infants >70 breaths/min; younger than 1 year old and children >50 breaths/min; or signs of distress)
• Toxic appearing
• Failure of outpatient treatment

The patient is transferred to the ED without complications. Chest radiography is done and shows consolidation in the left lower lobe.

Which of the following is the next most likely pathogen?

a. *Mycoplasma pneumoniae*

b. *Streptococcus pneumoniae*

c. Methicillin-resistant *Staphylococcus aureus* (MRSA)

d. *Haemophilus influenzae* type B (Hib)

Answer b. *Streptococcus pneumoniae*

The most common bacterial cause of pneumonia is streptococcal pneumonia. The other pathogens do cause pneumonia but are not the most likely. *Mycoplasma* does not lead to focal lobar consolidation. *Mycoplasma* has an envelope with no specific cell wall. The radiograph in mycoplasma looks just like viral pneumonia or pneumocystis.

MRSA and Hib are just not as statistically common as pneumococcus.

> *The patient is prescribed the proper antibiotics and improves. The patient is discharged home after 3 days.*

CASE 5: Foreign Body Aspiration

Setting: *ED*

CC: *"My child was choking and coughing."*

Vitals: *HR, 120 beats/min; RR, 21 breaths/min*

HPI: *A 2-year-old child presents to the ED for an episode of choking and coughing. The mother states that she turned her back to answer the phone for a second when the baby started to cough and gasp for air while playing with her older brother. A 5-year-old sibling states that the patient put a Lego in her mouth.*

Physical Exam:
- *Nothing visualized in the mouth*
- *Decreased breath sounds to right side*

Which of the following is the most accurate test of this patient?

a. ABG analysis

b. CXR

c. Bronchoscopy

d. Heimlich maneuver

Answer c. Bronchoscopy

Bronchoscopy is both diagnostic and therapeutic for patients with foreign body aspiration. ABG analysis will not diagnose or treat the aspiration; it will only give us information on the respiratory status of the patient. The best course of action will be to remove the foreign body so that the patient may breathe again. CXR may or may not show the object. If the object is radiolucent, CXR will be completely normal. Heimlich maneuver is contraindicated in patients who have a partial airway obstruction because the maneuver may actually cause the object to move and completely block the airway. The patient is currently coughing and gasping for air, so the airway is not completely blocked.

The patient needs oxygen, an oximeter or ABG, and CXR, but the most accurate of all of these is the bronchoscopy.

Think foreign body aspiration when a child is left alone and starts to cough.

Think of foreign body aspiration when there are persistent symptoms such as dyspnea, chronic cough, or recurring infections.

The patient undergoes bronchoscopy, and a blue Lego is retrieved from the right mainstem bronchus.

CASE 6: Cystic Fibrosis

Setting: *Office*

CC: *"My child hasn't passed stool."*

Vitals: *HR, 140 beats/min; RR, 30 breaths/min; weight, 5 lbs*

HPI: *A 2-day-old boy, born via normal spontaneous vaginal delivery at 39 weeks' gestation to a G_1P_0 white mother with a routine prenatal history, has not passed a stool yet. According to the mother, the patient's abdomen seems to be distended, and the patient vomited once. The vomit was green. The mother thought that it was normal for newborns to vomit.*

Physical Exam:
- *Alert, crying*
- *Heart sounds normal with no murmurs*
- *Lungs are clear to auscultation bilaterally*
- *Abdomen is distended*
- *Rectum is patent*

Abdominal Radiography Shows: *Bowel obstruction in the small bowel*

Which of the following is the most likely diagnosis of this patient?

a. Hirschsprung disease

b. Necrotizing enterocolitis (NEC)

c. Meconium ileus

d. Intussusception

e. Imperforate anus

Answer c. Meconium ileus

Meconium ileus presents in a newborn when the first stool (meconium) fails to pass and causes an obstruction in the intestines. This presents with abdominal distension, vomiting bilious materials, and failure of stool to pass. The abdominal radiography of meconium ileus shows an obstruction in the small intestines.

Hirschsprung disease is the failure of the nerves to innervate the last portions of the colon, leading to failure of meconium to pass in the first 48 hours of life. It also leads to abdominal distension and vomiting. However, abdominal radiography will show a thin last portion of the colon with a megacolon before it.

NEC will show pneumatosis intestinalis on abdominal radiography. The child will be feeding poorly, have temperature instability, and have bloody stool.

Intussusception usually occurs in children infants or toddlers who have intermittent abdominal pain that comes in 20- to 30-minute intervals. The patients will get into the fetal position to help relieve the obstruction. Target sign on abdominal radiography is pathognomonic. Imperforate anus was ruled out during the physical examination.

> *The patient is diagnosed with meconium ileus, and a nasogastric (NG) tube is placed without complications. After several days of NG tube and intravenous feedings, the patient improves.*

Which of the following is the next step in the diagnosis of this patient?

a. Sweat chloride testing

b. *CFTR* gene testing

c. Nasal potential difference

Answer a. Sweat chloride testing

All three tests are done to confirm cystic fibrosis (CF). However, the sweat chloride testing is the initial test of choice. The patient must be 2 weeks old and 4.4 lbs in weight for the test result to be reliable. Gene testing for mutations in the *CFTR* gene is done if the sweat chloride test result is positive or indeterminate. It is not done if the sweat chloride test result is negative. The nasal potential difference is done when the DNA and sweat chloride test results are inconclusive but the patient is exhibiting clinical signs of CF. Nasal potential difference measures electrodes placed in the nasal mucosa and looks at changes in response to difference nasal perfusion.

> *The patient had a sweat chloride test; the result was greater than 60 mmol/L. Two mutations on the CFTR gene were identified, one of which was a G551D mutation. The patient was diagnosed with CF.*

Mechanism of CF (Figure 4-3)
- Mutation in CF transmembrane conductance regulator (CFTR)
- Loss of flow of chloride and water across membranes
- No chloride or water flow = clogged lung, pancreas, and gastrointestinal tract
- *CFTR* on chromosome 7

Which of the following is the treatment of choice for CF patients with this gene mutation when older than 6 years old?

a. Albuterol

b. Inhaled DNase I

c. Ivacaftor

d. Azithromycin

Answer c. Ivacaftor

Ivacaftor is an oral drug that has been approved for use in children age 6 years and older with the *G551D* mutation (Figure 4-4). This medication restores the functioning of the

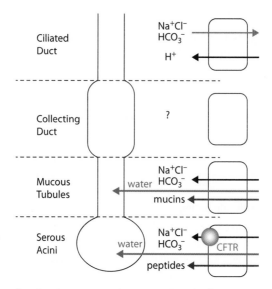

Figure 4-3. CFTR. (Used with permission from Conrad Fischer.)

mutant CF protein, allowing the medication to treat all of the related symptoms, not just the pulmonary symptoms. Albuterol is a bronchodilator that is used in an acute exacerbation. Azithromycin is a macrolide antibiotic and is indicated at the first sign of pulmonary complications. Inhaled DNase I decreases the viscosity of the sputum and should be used patients who have a daily cough.

> Patients with CF should receive yearly flu shots and the pneumococcal vaccination.

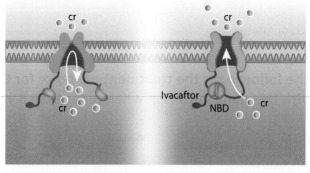

G551D Mutation - Class III gating defect   G551D Mutation defect reversed with ivacaftor

Figure 4-4. CFTR mutations. (Used with permission from Conrad Fischer.)

Mechanism of ivacaftor
• Addresses genetic defect in CF
• *G551D* mutation
• Amino acid glycine at position 551 replaced with aspartic acid
• Ivacaftor increases chloride transport through *CFTR*

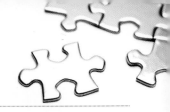

CHAPTER 5

EAR, NOSE, AND THROAT

CASE 1: Otitis Media

Setting: *Office*

CC: *"My ear hurts."*

Vitals: *T, 100.7°F; HR, 110 beats/min; RR, 25 breaths/min*

HPI: *A 4-year-old boy is brought to the office because he is tugging at his left ear. The mother states that for the past 4 days, the patient has been eating less, has been more irritable, and has been tugging on his left ear. The patient also had a low-grade fever that was resolved with acetaminophen. The patient has not been on antibiotics recently and has no allergies.*

Physical Exam:
- *Awake, alert, crying*
- *Left tympanic membrane is bulging and erythematous (Figure 5-1)*
- *Right tympanic membrane is erythematous*
- *Pharynx: Erythematous*
- *Heart sounds: Normal*
- *Lungs: Clear to auscultation bilaterally*

Which of the following is the treatment of choice for this patient?

a. Amoxicillin

b. Amoxicillin–clavulanate

c. Azithromycin

d. Cefdinir

e. Ceftriaxone

Answer a. Amoxicillin

Amoxicillin is the treatment of choice for acute otitis media. Amoxicillin–clavulanate is the first-line treatment if the patient had been on antibiotics recently or was at increased risk of β-lactam resistance. Azithromycin is used if the patient had an anaphylactic reaction when penicillin was taken. However, azithromycin does not kill *Haemophilus influenzae*, a common microbe that causes otitis media. Cefdinir is given to patients who had a rash in response to penicillin. Ceftriaxone is administered intramuscularly and may be given to patients who cannot tolerate oral medications or have severe infections.

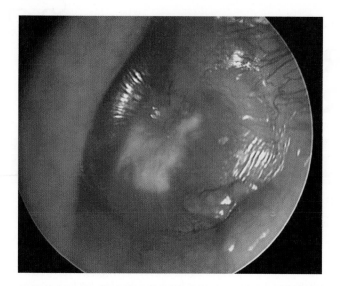

Figure 5-1. Bulging tympanic membrane. (Reproduced with permission from Wein RO, et al. Disorders of the head and neck. In: Brunicardi F, et al., eds. *Schwartz's Principles of Surgery.* 10th ed. New York, NY: McGraw-Hill; 2014. Fig. 18-1.)

> *The patient was given the treatment of choice and continued to have a fever after 72 hours on the antibiotics.*

Vitals: *T, 100.6°F; HR, 110 beats/min; RR, 22 breaths/min*

Physical Exam:
- *Awake, alert*
- *Left tympanic membrane is bulging and erythematous*
- *Right tympanic membrane is erythematous*
- *Pharynx: Erythematous*
- *Heart sounds: Normal*
- *Lungs: Clear to auscultation bilaterally*

Which of the following is the next step in the management of this patient?

a. Continue amoxicillin

b. Start amoxicillin–clavulanate

c. Start azithromycin

d. Start trimethoprim–sulfamethoxazole

Answer b. Start amoxicillin–clavulanate

The patient has failed treatment with amoxicillin alone as evidenced by a continued fever after 72 hours on antibiotics. Treatment failure is defined as a lack of improvement in 48 to

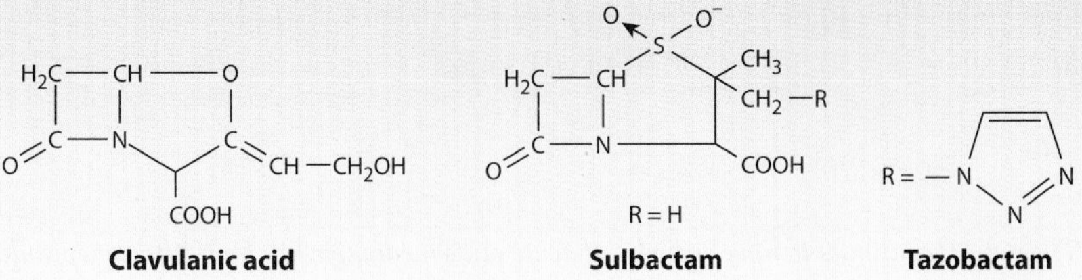

Figure 5-2. Molecular structure of antibiotics. (Reproduced with permission from Deck DH, Winston LG. Chapter 43. Beta-lactam & other cell wall- & membrane-active antibiotics. In: Katzung BG, Masters SB, Trevor AJ, eds. *Basic & Clinical Pharmacology.* 12th ed. New York, NY: McGraw-Hill; 2012.)

72 hours after the initiation of antibiotics. The treatment of choice for initial treatment failure is amoxicillin–clavulanate because it will increase the spectrum to kill the β-lactamase–producing bacteria. Other choices for treatment failure include cefdinir and ceftriaxone. Azithromycin and trimethoprim–sulfamethoxazole are not recommended in treatment failure because they do not cover *H. influenzae* (the most likely pathogen to cause treatment failure). If the patient has treatment failure, do NOT continue to give the same antibiotic.

The patient's acute otitis media resolves after administration of amoxicillin–clavulanate. However, in less than 1 month, the patient returns with acute otitis media.

Mechanism of antibiotics (Figure 5-2)
- Cell wall inhibitors: penicillin, cephalosporins, carbapenem, aztreonam
- Never act synergistically when used together because the mechanism is the same
- Clavulanic acid: inhibits β-lactamase; looks like β-lactam ring (Figure 5-2)

What is the next step in the management of this patient?

a. Amoxicillin

b. Amoxicillin–clavulanate

c. Azithromycin

d. Ceftriaxone

Answer e. Ceftriaxone

The patient most likely never completely cleared the infection from less than 30 days ago. Therefore, starting the same antibiotics (amoxicillin, amoxicillin–clavulanate) will not help. Azithromycin does not have broad-spectrum coverage. Ceftriaxone has broad-spectrum coverage and covers *Streptococcus pneumoniae*.

If the patient returned to the office more than 30 days after treatment for acute otitis media, then it would most likely be a new pathogen, and treatment with amoxicillin would be indicated.

Recurrence in <30 days = same pathogen
Recurrence in >30 days = different pathogen

The patient continues to have episodes of acute otitis media. He has four different episodes in less than 6 months.

Which of the following is the next step in the management of this patient?

a. Place on prophylactic amoxicillin   **c.** Place tympanostomy tubes
b. Place on prophylactic Cipro ear drops

Answer c. Place tympanostomy tubes

If patients have more than three episodes of acute otitis media in 6 months or four or more episodes in 1 year, it is an indication for tympanostomy tubes. Prophylactic antibiotics or ear drops are not recommended.

CASE 2: Otitis Externa

Setting: *Office*

CC: *"My ear hurts."*

Vitals: *T, 100.2°F; HR, 105 beats/min; RR, 20 breaths/min*

HPI: *A 7-year-old girl with no past medical history presents the office because her right ear has been hurting for 2 days. She states that it is dull and achy pain. The mother states that the patient has been irritable and had a low-grade temperature. The patient states that she woke up this morning with yellow stains on her pillowcase.*

Physical Exam:
- *Left ear: Tympanic membrane is normal*
- *Right ear: External ear canal slightly edematous; tympanic membrane partially obstructed because of canal swelling. Pain on movement of pinna. Cerumen present.*
- *Pharynx: Normal*
- *Heart sounds: Normal*
- *Lungs: Clear to auscultation bilaterally*

Which of the following is the most likely pathogen to be the cause?

a. Candida albicans

b. H. influenza

c. Streptococci

d. Pseudomonas

Answer d. Pseudomonas

All of the bacteria listed are possible causes of otitis externa; however, the most common cause is *Pseudomonas. Candida albicans* is most commonly found in elderly adults who use hearing aids.

Which of the following is the treatment of choice for this patient?

a. Ciprofloxacin–dexamethasone ear drops

b. Trimethoprim–sulfamethoxazole

c. Amoxicillin

Answer a. Ciprofloxacin–dexamethasone ear drops

Topical antibiotics are superior to oral antibiotics in otitis externa except during complications or immunosuppression. Ciprofloxacin–dexamethasone ear drops have both the antibiotic and antiinflammatory properties. The antiinflammatory properties should help with the pain.

Mechanism of quinolones
• Inhibition of DNA gyrase
• You cannot reproduce genetic material unless you unwind DNA.
• No DNA gyrase (topoisomerase) = no reproduction of DNA or RNA

CASE 3: Malignant Otitis Externa

Setting: *Office*

CC: *"My ear and head hurt."*

Vitals: *T, 101.4°F; HR, 125 beats/min; RR, 25 breaths/min*

HPI: *A 4-year-old boy is brought to the office with his mother for ear pain and headache. The mother states that the patient developed a fever 2 days ago for which she has been giving him acetaminophen and ibuprofen. She then noticed this morning that his right ear appeared red and was sticking out farther than the other ear. The patient has been pulling on the right ear, has been irritable, and has been eating less.*

Physical Exam:
- *Awake, alert, crying*
- *Right ear: Pinna slightly erythematous and farther away from skull when compared with left; ear canal edematous. Pain on palpation of right mastoid.*
- *Left ear: Normal; no pain on palpation of mastoid*
- *Heart sounds: Normal*
- *Lung sounds: Clear to auscultation*

Which of the following is the next step in the management of this patient?

a. Ciprofloxacin and dexamethasone ear drops

b. Complete blood count (CBC)

c. Computed tomography (CT) scan of the head

d. Amoxicillin

e. Biopsy

Answer c. Computed tomography (CT) scan of the head

This patient may have malignant otitis external. This is an infection and complication of otitis externa, when the infection moves into the mastoid process and can cause cranial osteomyelitis. An elevated white blood cell (WBC) count on the CBC is too nonspecific. The WBCs would be elevated in any infection. Imaging such as CT or magnetic resonance imaging (MRI) of the head is more specific. The next step for this patient would be transferring to the emergency department (ED) for a head CT and to begin treatment. Antibiotics should not be started without a diagnosis.

Although biopsy is the most accurate test, it should not be done until after a CT or MRI of the mastoid air cells.

> The patient is transferred to the emergency department. The patient is found to have an elevated WBC count, elevated erythrocyte sedimentation rate (ESR), and elevated C-reactive protein (CRP). The patient's head CT shows edema surrounding the right mastoid process and bone erosion.

Which of the following is the best therapy for this patient?

a. Amoxicillin

b. Amoxicillin–clavulanate

c. Azithromycin

d. Ceftazidime

e. Clindamycin

Answer d. Ceftazidime

Ceftazidime is an antipseudomonal drug that is often used in children with malignant otitis externa. First-line treatment in patients older than the age of 18 years is ciprofloxacin. The treatment, as with all forms of osteomyelitis, should last 6 to 8 weeks if surgical debridement is not done.

The medications of that adequately cover gram-negative bacilli are the following:

• Fluoroquinolones
• Carbapenems
• Piperacillin, ticarcillin
• Third and fourth generation cephalosporins
• Aztreonam

CASE 4: Strep Throat

Setting: *Office*

CC: *"My throat hurts."*

Vitals: *T, 101.1°F; HR, 110 beats/min*

HPI: *A 7-year-old girl is brought to the office after 2 days of sore throat, fever, and chills. The patient states that the sore throat is located on both sides. The mother states that the child had a fever with a temperature maximum of 102.3°F. The patient has also complained of abdominal pain with nausea.*

Physical Exam:
- *Awake, alert, oriented*
- *Bilateral tympanic membranes: Normal*
- *Pharynx is erythematous and enlarged with exudates*
- *Petechial lesions seen on palate*
- *Cervical lymph node enlargement is present bilaterally*

Which of the following is the most likely cause of this infection?

a. Influenza type A

b. Group A streptococcus

c. *Neisseria gonorrhea*

e. *Corynebacterium diphtheriae*

Answer b. Group A Streptococcus

Group A streptococcus is the most common pathogen with these symptoms and physical examination findings. One point should be given to the following criteria:
- Abscense of cough
- Swollen or tender anterior cervical lymph nodes
- Temp >100.4
- Tonsillar exudates or swelling
- Age 3-14 years old
- No points for age 15–44 years old negative 1 point for age 44+

A score of 4 points or more, the patient likely has group A streptococcus and should be treated empirically. Influenza type A is characterized by a high fever, body aches, cough, and headache.

N. gonorrhea infection is uncommon, but it should be included in the differential diagnosis in sexually active adolescents. If the examination wants you to choose this answer, it will give you a hint!

C. diphtheriae is common in undeveloped countries but not in the United States. Diphtheria causes pharyngitis with mild erythema. However, as it progresses, a gray membrane covers the throat and mucous membranes.

Which of the following is the next best step in the management of this patient?

a. Rapid strep test

b. Heterophile antibody testing

c. ASO testing

d. Streptokinase

Answer a. Rapid strep test

The rapid strep test is easily done in the office. This is a swab of the throat, and results are ready in about 5 minutes. The rapid strep test should be performed on patients with a clinical score of 5 or more. A throat culture is the most accurate, but because the results will not be ready for more than 48 hours, a rapid test should be done. The throat culture should still be performed on patients with a negative rapid test result. The ASO and streptokinase testing are blood tests that are based on antibodies to streptococci. These test results generally will not be positive for 3 weeks after the initial infection.

The heterophile antibody testing is done to rule out infectious mononucleosis or Epstein-Barr virus (EBV). EBV should be considered in patients who have persistent symptoms or general lymphadenopathy or develop a rash after treatment for strep with penicillin.

A rapid strep test is done, and the result is positive.

Which of the following is the next step in the management of this patient?

a. Amoxicillin

b. Clindamycin

c. Doxycycline

d. Trimethoprim–sulfamethoxazole

Answer a. Amoxicillin

Amoxicillin is the first-line treatment in patients with strep throat. If the patient is allergic to penicillin, macrolides or cephalosporins are the first-line treatment. Trimethoprim–sulfamethoxazole and the tetracyclines are not recommended in patients with strep throat.

The patient is given amoxicillin and improves rapidly. The 10-day course is completed.

CASE 5: Peritonsilar Abscess

Setting: *Office*

CC: *"My child has a sore throat and trouble swallowing."*

Vitals: *T, 101.5°F; HR, 120 beats/min; RR, 25 breaths/min*

HPI: *A 7-year-old boy was brought to the office for a unilateral sore throat and trouble swallowing for 2 days. The patient has been complaining of an itchy throat for the past week, but the patient was not brought to the doctor. The patient now is having severe pain on the right tonsil with right ear pain for 2 days. The patient has also had decreased oral intake and pain while swallowing.*

Physical Exam:
- *Awake, alert, oriented*
- *Muffled voice*
- *Enlarged right side tonsil with deviation of the uvula to the left side*
- *Lungs: Clear to auscultation bilaterally*
- *Heart sounds: Normal*

Which of the following is the most likely diagnosis of this patient?

a. Tonsillitis

b. Epiglottitis

c. Pharyngeal abscess

d. Retropharyngeal abscess

Answer c. Pharyngeal abscess

Pharyngeal abscess is the most common deep infection in the neck, characterized by unilateral sore throat, muffled voice, drooling, and neck and ear pain on the affected side. Epiglottitis has most often been from *Hemophilus influenzae*. Epiglottitis is now rare because of vaccination of children. We vaccinate children @ 2, 4, 6 months of age to prevent this deadly disease. Epiglottitis is inconsistent with this presentation because it is rapidly progressive with cough and respiratory distress. Retropharyngeal abscess usually presents with neck stiffness and no tonsillar findings. Tonsillitis is usually bilateral.

Change the setting to the ED.

What is the next step in the management of this patient?

a. CBC

b. Throat culture

c. CT of the neck

d. Biopsy

e. Rapid strep test

Answer c. CT of the neck

As long as the child is stable and not in respiratory distress, CT of the neck can distinguish between an abscess and cellulitis. However, no actual testing is necessary to make the diagnosis. The physical examination could make the diagnosis alone.

> CT is done and shows a collection of fluid with a ring around the collection.

Which of the following is the treatment of choice?

a. Levofloxacin   **c.** Incision and drainage
b. Clindamycin   **d.** Intubation

Answer c. Incision and drainage

The fluid-filled mass with a ring is an abscess. The only treatment for an abscess is incision and drainage followed by antibiotics. However, if the abscess is not drained, the antibiotics will not work. The fluid should be collected and sent for culture. While awaiting culture results, ampicillin–sulbactam should be administered. Clindamycin is a possible choice if the patient is allergic to penicillin. Intubation may be necessary if the patient is in respiratory distress.

Incision and drainage provides the fastest relief of symptoms. Clindamycin and quinolones are the wrong choice in antibiotics.

> The patient goes for incision and drainage, and 10 cc of purulent material is expelled and sent for culture.

CASE 6: Retinoblastoma

Setting: *Office*

CC: *"My baby needs to have his 1-month shots."*

Vitals: *T, 98.1°F; HR, 140 beats/min; RR, 30 breaths/min; weight, 8 lb*

HPI: *A 1-month-old boy is brought to the office for his 1-month visit. The patient is being breastfed by his mother, gaining weight, opening his eyes more, and smiling. The mother has no concerns.*

Physical Exam:
- *Awake, crying*
- *White reflex is present in the right eye; red reflex is present in left eye*
- *Tympanic membranes: Normal bilaterally*
- *Pharynx: Injected*
- *Lungs: Clear to auscultation bilaterally*
- *Heart sounds: Normal*
- *Abdomen: Soft, nondistended*
- *Hips: Barlow and Ortolani negative*
- *Skin: No rashes are noted*

Which of the following is the next step in the management of this patient?

a. Administer the diphtheria, tetanus, and pertussis (DTap) vaccination
b. Administer the rotavirus vaccine
c. Referral to ophthalmology
d. Referral to surgery
e. Continue to monitor and have patient return at 2 months of age

Answer c. Refer to ophthalmology

The child has a white reflex on eye examination, indicating the child has retinoblastoma. Retinoblastoma is the most common intraocular malignancy of childhood, and the child could lose his vision and possibly his life if left untreated. The next step in management is prompt referral to an ophthalmologist.

General surgery is not the right specialty. Hepatitis B vaccination is given at 1 month of age. DTap and rotavirus vaccines are given starting at 2 months of age. Monitoring of the patient is wasting precious time. Even if you are unsure if the reflex is white, refer to ophthalmology.

The patient is diagnosed with retinoblastoma.

Which of the following is a risk factor for retinoblastoma?

a. Congenital rubella   **c.** Family history

b. Congenital varicella

Answer c. Family history

Family history is the strongest risk factor for retinoblastoma. Children who have had a parent or sibling with retinoblastoma are at high risk. Patients with a family history of retinoblastoma should be evaluated by an ophthalmologist after birth, then every 3 to 4 months until the child is 4 years old, and then every 6 months until 6 years old. Genetic testing for these patients is also available for the retinoblastoma genes on 13q14 deletion. Congenital rubella causes cataracts, which is a cloudy white appearance in the eye. Congenital varicella may also cause cataracts or nystagmus.

Retinoblastoma syndrome
• Deletion in 13q14

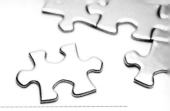

CHAPTER **6**

ENDOCRINOLOGY

CASE 1: **Hypothyroid**

Setting: *Office*

CC: *"My baby's newborn screen was abnormal."*

Vitals: *T, 98.9°F; HR, 140s; RR, 35 breaths/min; weight, 9 lb*

HPI: *A mother brought her 4-week-old son to the office for his 1-month check up. The mother states that the baby is eating well, sleeping 3 to 4 hours at a time, and is smiling. The mother is concerned because the state notified her that there was something abnormal on the child's newborn screening with the thyroid. The mother is unsure what it is and did not bring the record.*

Physical Exam:
- *Awake, alert, eyes open, + red reflex*
- *Tympanic membranes: Normal bilaterally*
- *Pharynx: Normal*
- *+ Red reflex bilaterally*
- *Lungs: Clear to auscultation*
- *Heart sounds: Normal*
- *Abdomen: Soft, nondistended*

Which of the following is the next step in the management of this patient?

a. Monitor and return in 1 month

b. Thyroid profile (thyroxine [T_4], thyroid-stimulating hormone [TSH] levels)

c. Thyroid ultrasonography

d. Growth hormone level

e. Insulinlike growth factor (IGF) level

Answer b. Thyroid profile (thyroxine [T_4], thyroid-stimulating hormone [TSH] levels)

The patient had an abnormal thyroid on the newborn screening. Thyroid abnormalities are most common preventable cause of mental retardation. Thyroid ultrasonography may be needed after the thyroid profile. Not acting on the information and continuing to monitor the patient are incorrect. Most newborns are asymptomatic at birth.

Symptoms of congenital hypothyroidism
- Lethargy
- Hoarse cry
- Feeding problems
- Macroglossia
- Large fontanels
- Hypotonia
- Hypothermia
- Jaundice

Thyroid abnormalities are the most common *preventable* cause of mental retardation.

Newborns are often asymptomatic because maternal thyroid hormones cross the placenta.

Mechanism of developmental defects in hypothyroidism
- Thyroxine is needed for neural growth.
- No thyroid hormone = brain permanently nonworking
- Thyroid hormone needed for growth hormone release
- No thyroid hormone = no growth

The patient's thyroid profile returns with a T_4 level less than 10 ng/dL and TSH of 30 mlU/L.

Which of the following is the most likely diagnosis?

a. Primary hypothyroidism
b. Subclinical hypothyroidism
c. Central hypothyroidism

Answer a. Primary hypothyroidism

Primary hypothyroidism is characterized by a low T_4 level and high TSH level. Subclinical hypothyroidism is normal T_4 level and high TSH level. Central hypothyroidism is a low T_4 level with a normal TSH level.

Primary hypothyroidism: low T_4; high TSH
Subclinical hypothyroidism: normal T_4; high TSH
Central hypothyroidism: low T_4; normal TSH

Which of the following is the next step in the management of this patient?

a. Treat with levothyroxine

b. Treat with methimazole

c. Serum thyroglobulin assay

d. Thyroid antibody testing

Answer a. Treat with levothyroxine

The treatment for hypothyroidism is levothyroxine. Methimazole is used to treat hyperthyroidism. Additional testing may be done in some cases, but it does not alter the treatment. Therefore, in the effort to prevent mental retardation, start treatment.

Thyroid hormone is essential for normal brain development of babies!

CASE 2: Diabetes

Setting: *Office*

CC: *"My child has been complaining of abdominal pain and has been urinating a lot."*

Vitals: *T, 98.9°F; HR, 90 beats/min; RR, 25 breaths/min*

HPI: *A 4-year-old boy with no past medical history presents to the office with his mother for abdominal pain and an increase in urinary frequency for the past week. The mother states that for the past week, she seems to be taking him to the bathroom more frequently. The mother states that this morning, he started complaining of abdominal pain that is generalized and severe.*

Physical Exam:
- *Awake and alert*
- *Tympanic membranes: Bilaterally normal*
- *Pharynx: No erythema or edema of tonsils*
- *Lungs: Clear to auscultation bilaterally*
- *Heart sounds: Normal*
- *Abdomen: Soft, nontender, nondistended; positive bowel sounds*

Which of the following is the next step in the management of this patient?

a. Complete blood count (CBC)

b. Computed tomography (CT) of the abdomen

c. Complete metabolic profile (CMP)

d. Urinalysis (UA)

Answer d. Urinalysis (UA)

The patient has symptoms of urinary frequency. Urinary frequency can be associated with several diagnoses, and UA is an easy test that can be done in the office with immediate results. A CBC and CMP are blood tests that will take several hours to return. CT of the abdomen will be able to identify any organ or structural abnormalities, but not all of the differential diagnoses are seen on CT.

UA returned with greater than 1000 mg/dL of glucose, and negative for ketones, leukocytes, nitrates, blood, and protein.

Which of the following is the next step in the management of this patient?

a. Fingerstick glucose

b. Oral glucose tolerance test (OGTT)

c. Metformin

d. Insulin

Answer a. Fingerstick glucose

A fingerstick can and should be done in the office as soon as a UA is positive for glucose. One of the diagnostic criteria for diabetes is a random glucose level more than 200 mg/dL with symptoms of hyperglycemia (polyuria and polydipsia). This test alone can diagnose diabetes at this time. An OGTT can also diagnose diabetes, but a fingerstick is the next best step. Administering medications is not recommended until a definitive diagnosis is made.

Mechanism of polyuria in diabetes (Figure 6-1)
- Sodium-glucose linked transporter (SGLT) receptors in the proximal tubule begin to saturate at glucose >200 mg/dL.
- When SGLT receptors saturate, glucose spills into urine.
- When fully saturated at glucose level 350 mg/dL, there is osmotic diuresis with glucose spilling into urine pulling water with it.
- Increased drinking (polydipsia) and eating (polyphagia) result.

Diagnostic criteria for diabetes
- HgbA1c >6.5% mg/dL
- Two fasting glucose >126 mg/dL
- Random glucose >200 mg/dL with symptoms
- Positive OGTT result

The fingerstick returns with a glucose level of 450 mg/dL. The patient is diagnosed with type I diabetes.

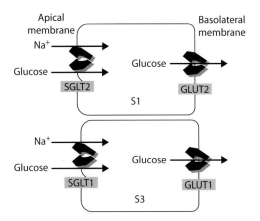

Figure 6-1. Glucose transport. (Reproduced with permission from Conrad Fischer.)

Which of the following is the goal of treatment?

a. HgbA1c <7.0

b. HgbA1c <7.5

c. HgbA1c <8

d. HgbA1c <8.5

Answer d. HgbA1c <8.5

HgbA1C is a measurement of the average of blood glucoses over a 3-month period. If the HgbA1C is low, there is a higher risk of hypoglycemia in children. In children, one needs to balance the risk of hypoglycemia and risk of severe hypoglycemia with the benefits of glycemic control. Tight control leads to episodes of hypoglycemia. Hypoglycemia is very damaging to a developing child's brain. Mild hyperglycemia is less dangerous than hypoglycemia.

Children are treated with insulin regiments and often insulin pumps. No oral medications are indicated in type I diabetes.

Age-based goals for HgbA1C:
• Age younger than 6 years: <8.5%
• Ages 6 to 12 years: <8%
• Ages 13 to 19 years: <7.5%
• Age 19 years and older: <7%.

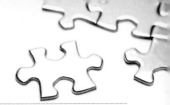

CHAPTER **7**

POISONING

CASE 1: Acetaminophen

Setting: *ED*

CC: *"My child took acetaminophen."*

HPI: *A 3-year-old girl is brought to the emergency department for ingestion of an unknown amount of acetaminophen. The mother states that the girl was left home with the grandmother, who fell asleep on the couch. When the grandmother woke up, she found the child playing with a bottle of acetaminophen with multiple pills on the floor. There was an unknown number of pills in the bottle and an unknown number ingested. The grandmother found her more than an hour ago; an exact time of ingestion is unknown, but less than 2 hours is suspected. The patient currently has no symptoms.*

Physical Exam: *Within normal limits*

Which of the following is the next step in the management of this patient?

a. Activated charcoal

b. Intubation

c. Gastric lavage

d. Emergent dialysis

Answer a. Activated charcoal

Children who may have a toxic ingestion of acetaminophen should receive activated charcoal if the event occurs less than 4 hours after the ingestion. Intubation is not needed in patients who can protect their airways. There is no indication that the child cannot protect her airway. If the test wants you to know the answer, it has to tell you something! Gastric lavage is not indicated in adults or children because there is a high rate of aspiration. Activated charcoal is more effective with fewer risks. Emergency dialysis is not indicated as initial management.

The proper medication is administered, and labs are drawn.

Which of the following is the treatment of choice for toxicity?

a. *N*-acetylcysteine

b. Dimercaprol

c. Deferoxamine

d. Glucagon

e. Octreotide

Answer a. *N*-acetylcysteine

All of the answers are antidotes for a specific type of poisoning:

Antidotes

Poisoning	Antidote
Acetaminophen	*N*-acetylcysteine
Heavy metal poisoning	Dimercaprol
Iron poisoning	Deferoxamine
Beta-blocker or calcium channel blocker	Glucagon
Oral sulfonylurea poisoning	Octreotide

> *The child is administered the antidote, and the acetaminophen level, international normalized ratio, and liver enzymes are monitored. The patient never develops abnormalities of the liver enzymes.*

Mechanism of acetylcysteine
- Prodrug of L-cysteine
- Produces biologic antioxidant glutathione
- Glutathione blocks oxidant damage from acetaminophen metabolites

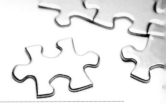

CHAPTER 8

ORTHOPEDICS

CASE 1: A Loud Clunk

Setting: *Office*

CC: *"I am here for follow-up."*

Vitals: *Stable*

HPI: *A 1-week-old girl is brought to the office by her mother for follow-up. The child was born preterm at 32 weeks' gestation in the breech condition but has had an unremarkable course since discharge. The patient's older brother was born with "hip problems" as per the mother.*

Physical Exam: *A palpable "clunk" is present when the hip is directed in and out of the acetabulum.*

What is the most likely diagnosis?

a. Developmental dysplasia of the hip (DDH)

b. Legg-Calvé-Perthes disease (LCPD)

c. Slipped capital femoral epiphysis (SCFE)

Answer a. Developmental dysplasia of the hip (DDH)

DDH presents in preterm children, more commonly in girls with breeching positioning in utero, with a family history and pathognomonic tests on physical examination. The two findings are known as the Barlow and Ortolani's tests. Whereas LCPD is more commonly seen in adolescents, SCFE is seen in young obese teenagers.

DDH was previously called congenital dysplasia of the hip.

On USMLE Step 3, the answer to which hip condition is affecting the child is almost entirely based on age.

Barlow sign is when a clunk is felt as the hip subluxates out of the acetabulum.

Ortolani sign is referred to as a clunk felt when the hip reduces into the acetabulum, with the hip in abduction.

The growth of the acetabulum depends on ossification of the pubis, ilium, and ischium.

What is the best diagnostic test for this condition?

a. Radiography of the hip

b. Computed tomography (CT) scan of the hip

c. Ultrasonography of the affected hip

d. Ultrasonography of both hips

Answer d. Ultrasonography of both hips

The best diagnostic for a patient suspected of having DDH is ultrasonography of both hips. Radiography is the best test in a patient after 4 months of age. A CT scan would be far too much radiation and thus "too invasive" compared with simple ultrasonography. Ultrasonography of only one hip is incorrect because many patients have bilateral involvement.

Orders:
- *Ultrasonography of the bilateral hips*
- *Send the patient home.*
- *Have the patient return to the office in 2 days.*

Turn the clock forward.

Ultrasonography reveals dislocation of the hip joint bilaterally consistent with DDH given the patient's age.

What is the most appropriate therapy for this condition?

a. Pavlik harness

b. Bone pinning

c. Surgery with casts

d. Observation

e. Closed reduction

Answer a. Pavlik harness

The most appropriate therapy for a child with DDH is a Pavlik harness (Figure 8-1) for the first year of life. If the child does not improve, then surgical reduction and casting are the next steps in management.

The most common long-term complication of DDH is acetabular dysplasia.

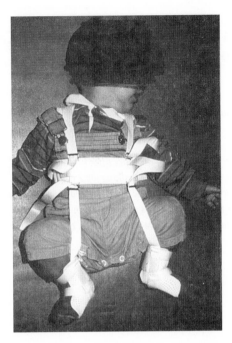

Figure 8-1. The Pavlik harness, a device used for treatment of hip dislocation, subluxation, and dysplasia. (Reproduced with permission from Rab GT. Chapter 10. Pediatric orthopedic surgery. In: Skinner HB, McMahon PJ, eds. *Current Diagnosis & Treatment in Orthopedics*. 5th ed. New York, NY: McGraw-Hill; 2014.)

Orders:
- *Pavlik harness*
- *Physical therapy*

Turn the clock forward, and the case will end.

If the case does not end, bring the patient back in 2 months, and if there is no improvement, order a surgical consult. Note that this will likely be the case if the child is close to 10 to 12 months of age.

CASE 2: Can't Run or Climb a Tree But Can See and Pee

Setting: *Office*

CC: *"My son's leg hurts."*

Vitals: *Stable*

HPI: *A 6-year-old boy is brought to the office after his father noticed he has been limping. The child states that he has had trouble walking for 2 months, but in the past 2 weeks, the difficulty is also associated with pain. The pain at its worst is 8 of 10, and the child says it is located to the front of his thigh. He says when he doesn't play outside, he rests, and he feels better. The parents say he did not have a fall, trauma, or sports-related accident.*

ROS:
- *No fevers*
- *No chills*
- *No recent illnesses*
- *No sick contacts*

Physical Exam:
- *Pain with passive range of motion*
- *Quadriceps muscle atrophy*
- *Antalgic gait noted on walking*

What is the most likely diagnosis?

a. Developmental dysplasia of the hip (DDH)

b. Legg-Calvé-Perthes disease (LCPD)

c. Slipped capital femoral epiphysis (SCFE)

Answer b. Legg-Calvé-Perthes disease (LCPD)

LCPD is characterized by a painless limp in a boy between the ages of 4 and 10 years. The etiology of the problem is related to osteonecrosis of the proximal femoral epiphysis and is thought to result from vascular compromise. SCFE is seen in young obese teenagers and presents with groin and knee pain. DDH is seen in infants several days after birth up to 1 year of age.

The pain of LCPD is referred to the groin, ipsilateral knee, or both.

What is the best diagnostic test for this condition?

a. Radiography of the hip
b. CT scan of the hip
c. Ultrasonography of the affected hip

d. Biopsy
e. DEXA or bone densitometry

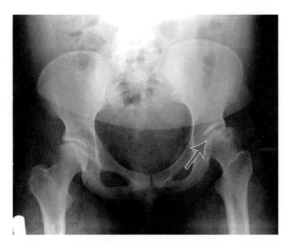

Figure 8-2. Legg-Calvé-Perthes disease. Chronic and significant deformity of the left femoral head is apparent. (Reproduced with permission from Hopkins-Mann C, Ogunnaike-Joseph D, Moro-Sutherland D. Chapter 133. Musculoskeletal disorders in children. In: Tintinalli JE, et al., eds. *Tintinalli's Emergency Medicine: A Comprehensive Study Guide.* 7th ed. New York, NY: McGraw-Hill; 2011.)

Answer a. Radiography of the hip

Radiography of the hip is the next best step management and the best diagnostic test for LCPD. Narrowing of the femoral head with compression and deformity of the femoral neck may occur as a result of vascular insufficiency. All other imaging modalities either expose the child to excessive radiation or lack the sensitivity for making the diagnosis.

Orders:
• *Radiography of the hip*

Radiography of the hip demonstrates compression collapse and lateral extrusion of the femoral head consistent with LCPD (Figure 8-2).

What is the most appropriate therapy for this condition?

a. Casting
b. Bed rest
c. Physical therapy

d. Surgical correction
e. All of the above

Answer e. All of the above

There is most appropriate therapy for LCPD, and the patient will need a hip replacement later in life. The therapies to increase mobility include casting, rest, and physical therapy. If the patient does not improve, surgery is indicated.

Orders:

• *Surgical consult*
• *Physical therapy*

Turn the clock forward, and the case will end.

CASE 3: My Leg Hurts

Setting: *Office*

CC: *"My hip hurts."*

Vitals: *Stable*

HPI: *A 14-year-old boy presents with left hip pain and knee pain. The child is obese and has been battling weight loss for 2 years. He has recently developed glucose intolerance because of his weight and wishes to begin an exercise regimen.*

ROS:
- *No fevers*
- *No chills*
- *No trauma*

Physical Exam:
- *External rotations and abduction are present with gentle passive hip flexion.*
- *Internal rotation is decreased and painful.*
- *An altered or "antalgic" gait is seen.*

What is the most likely diagnosis?

a. DDH

b. LCPD

c. SCFE

Answer c. SCFE

SCFE is the most likely diagnosis in adolescent boys who present with hip and knee pain in the setting of obesity. SCFE represents a unique type of instability of the proximal femoral growth plate from stress caused by shear forces from obesity. The fracture occurs at the hypertrophic zone of the physeal cartilage. Stress on the hip causes the epiphysis to move posteriorly and medially.

SCFE is more common in boys and occurs more commonly in the left hip.

Knee pain may be referred pain from the hip via the obturator nerve.

What is the next step in the management of this patient?

a. Radiography of the hip

b. Radiography of the femur

c. Radiography of the pelvis

d. Radiography of the entire body

Answer c. Radiography of the pelvis

The diagnosis requires radiography of the pelvis, including frog-leg lateral views. The head of the femur will appear like a "melting ice cream cone." This means blurring of the junction between the metaphysis and the growth plate. The purpose behind looking at the pelvis rather than the affected hip is that in about 20% of all cases, SCFE is present bilaterally at the time of presentation. CT is not better than radiography. Magnetic resonance imaging (MRI) should not be done first.

Orders:

• *Radiography of the hip*

Radiography of the pelvis shows bilateral melting ice cream cone signs consistent with SCFE.

As widening and slipping occur, the femoral neck rotates anteriorly while the head remains in the acetabulum.

What is the most appropriate therapy for this condition?

a. Bed rest   **c.** Physical therapy
b. Observation   **d.** Surgical correction

Answer d. Surgical correction

Surgical pinning with open or closed reduction is the most appropriate therapy for a patient with SCFE. Bed and observation can lead to complications and further breakdown of the hip joint. Physical therapy is adjunctive to the treatment of SCFE but is not the best intervention.

The most common complications of SCFE are osteonecrosis and chondrolysis.

Orders:

• *Surgical consult*
• *Physical therapy*

Turn the clock forward, and the case will end.

CASE 4: My Knee Hurts

Setting: *Office*

CC: *"My knee hurts."*

Vitals: *Stable*

HPI: *A 15-year-old male soccer player presents with swelling and pain over his right knee. He says he feels like his right knee is bigger than his left knee. He says he can't wear his shin guards up to his knees because touching the knee hurts.*

ROS:
- *No trauma*
- *No fevers*
- *No chills*

Physical Exam:
- *Prominence of tibial tubercle*
- *Swelling over the tibial tubercle*
- *Tender to palpation over the right tubercle with no pain on the left*
- *Normal range of motion*
- *No effusion*
- *Negative Lachman test result*

What is the most likely diagnosis?

a. Osgood-Schlatter disease (OSD)
b. Meniscus tear
c. Osteomyelitis
d. Anterior cruciate ligament (ACL) tear

Answer a. Osgood-Schlatter disease (OSD)

OSD is the most likely diagnosis in a patient with a stable knee that has pain over the tibial tubercle. The cause of OSD is repeated knee extension leading to microavulsions of the tibial tubercle. Whereas a tear in the meniscus usually develops after trauma to the knee and presents with locking of the knee, an ACL tear would have a positive Lachman test result. Osteomyelitis presents with fevers, erythema, and signs of systemic infection.

What is the next best step in the management of this patient?

a. Radiography of the knee
b. MRI of the knee
c. Physical therapy and rest
d. Steroid injections

Answer c. Physical therapy and rest

Imaging studies and laboratory tests are not required to make a diagnosis of OSD. Steroid injections are always the wrong answer. Steroid injections may make the insertion of the tendons weaker. Physical therapy, rest, and knee immobilization will improve symptoms. Patients normally have complete relief of symptoms in 12 to 24 months.

Orders:
- *Physical therapy*
- *Send the patient home*

Turn the clock forward, and the case will end.

CASE 5: **Another Broken Bone?**

Setting: *ED*

CC: *"He won't stop crying and won't listen to me."*

Vitals: *HR, 200 beats/min; RR, 30 breaths/min; BP, 90/45 mm Hg*

HPI: *A 3-year-old boy is brought into the emergency department after falling down while playing in the sandbox. The child has pain in his right arm and is holding it close to him. The child doesn't pay attention when you ask him questions. This child has been seen several times before for other fractures. The parents have been seen by child protective services because of the large number of posttraumatic injuries. Their findings are conclusive that the children are in a safe home.*

Physical Exam:
- *The right forearm is swollen and malformed.*
- *Bruising over the lower extremities*
- *Bluish tint to sclerae (Figure 8-3)*
- *Short stature*

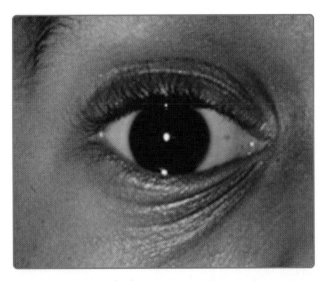

Figure 8-3. Osteogenesis imperfecta (OI). Blue sclerae are the most characteristic mucocutaneous feature of patients with mild OI. (Reproduced with permission from Dyer JA. Chapter 137. Lipoid proteinosis and heritable disorders of connective tissue. In: Goldsmith LA, et al., eds. *Fitzpatrick's Dermatology in General Medicine.* 8th ed. New York, NY: McGraw-Hill; 2012. eFigure 137-11.1.)

What is the most likely diagnosis?

a. Child abuse
b. Osteogenesis imperfecta (OI)

c. Lead poisoning
d. Osteopenia

Answer b. Osteogenesis imperfecta (OI)

OI is the most likely diagnosis when a young child presents with repeated fractures caused by fragile bones, blue sclerae, and early deafness. It can present in young children. Child abuse must be ruled out in patients who have recurrent fractures to ensure these children are not being physically hurt. Lead poisoning usually is stunted growth, and the patient will present with abdominal pain and neurologic dysfunction. Osteopenia is usually seen in elderly patients and is pre-osteoporosis.

> OI is an autosomal dominant inherited disorder.

> Type I collagen fibers are found in the bones, cornea, sclera, tendons, and dermis.

What is the most accurate test for the diagnosis of OI?

a. Calcium level
b. Anticollagen antibodies
c. Skeletal survey

d. Collagen synthesis analysis
from skin biopsy

Answer d. Collagen synthesis analysis from skin biopsy

The most accurate test for OI is to obtain a skin biopsy for collagen synthesis analysis by culturing dermal fibroblasts. Most laboratory values, including the calcium level, will be normal in OI, and there is no such thing as anticollagen antibodies. A skeletal survey is the best initial test, but because this child has been seen before and cleared by child protective services, you can assume a skeletal survey was done.

> OI is inherited in genes that codify for type I procollagen. The genes are *COL1A1* and *COL1A2*.

What is the next best step in the management of this patient?

a. Start pamidronate
b. Physical therapy

c. Fracture management
d. All of the above

Answer d. All of the above

There is no cure for OI, and therapy is aimed at fracture management, increasing bone mass, and correction of deformities from fractures. Oral bisphosphonates do not work, and thus infusions such as pamidronate are indicated.

> **Orders:**
> - *Physical therapy*
> - *Radiography*
> - *Pamidronate*
>
> *Turn the clock forward, and the case will end.*

CASE 6: Sunburst or Onions

Setting: *Office*

CC: *"My child's leg hurts."*

Vitals: *Stable*

HPI: *An 11-year-old boy presents with a painful lump in his leg, fevers, and weight loss over the past 6 months. His mother states that he no longer wishes to play outside with his friends because of the pain. Previous laboratory analysis reveals that his vitamin D levels are within normal limits. His mother denies any recent trauma or accidents.*

ROS:
- *No nausea*
- *Fevers*
- *Night sweats*
- *15-lb weight loss*

PE: *Painful lump over left lateral femur*

What is the next best step in the management of this patient?

a. Radiography of the femur

b. CT scan of the femur

c. MRI of the femur

d. Discharge home

Answer a. Radiography of the femur

Radiography of the femur is the best initial test for any child presenting with a painful localized lump and constitutional symptoms of malignancy. The classic finding on radiography is an onion-skin pattern (Figure 8-4) due to lytic lesions causing laminar periosteal elevation. CT, MRI, and discharge are not the best initial tests.

> The most accurate test for Ewing's sarcoma is analysis for a translocation t(11;22) via bone biopsy.

What is the most likely diagnosis?

a. Osteogenic sarcoma

b. Ewing's sarcoma

c. Osteoid osteoma

d. Rickets

Answer b. Ewing's sarcoma

Ewing's sarcoma is the most common cause of localized bone pain in a young child without history of trauma in the setting of fevers night sweats and weight loss. The classic finding of an onion-skin pattern due to lytic lesions causing laminar periosteal elevation is seen in Ewing's sarcoma.

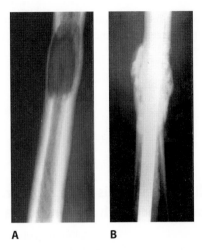

A   **B**

Figure 8-4. Ewing's sarcoma seen in the femur. (Reproduced with permission from Randall R, Ward R, Hoang BH. Chapter 5. Musculoskeletal oncology. In: Skinner HB, McMahon PJ, eds. *Current Diagnosis & Treatment in Orthopedics.* 5th ed. New York, NY: McGraw-Hill; 2014.)

What is the most likely diagnosis if the radiographs show a sunburst pattern (Figure 8-5)?

a. Osteogenic sarcoma   **c.** Osteoid osteoma
b. Ewing's sarcoma   **d.** Rickets

Answer a. Osteogenic sarcoma

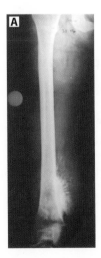
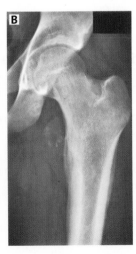
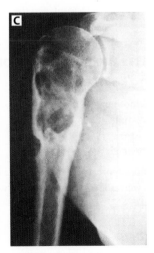

Figure 8-5. Sunburst pattern seen in the Osteogenic Sarcoma. (Reproduced with permission from Conley A, et al. Chapter 40. Soft tissue and bone sarcomas. In: Kantarjian HM, Wolff RA, Koller CA, eds. *The MD Anderson Manual of Medical Oncology.* 2nd ed. New York, NY: McGraw-Hill; 2011.)

Osteogenic sarcoma, which occurs more commonly in the second decade of life, is characterized by sclerotic destruction causing a "sunburst" appearance. Therapy includes chemotherapy and ablative surgery.

> **Orders:**
> • *If the diagnosis is osteogenic sarcoma, order an oncology consult and surgical consult.*
>
> *Turn the clock forward, and the case will end.*

What is the most likely diagnosis if the radiographs show a small round central lucency with a sclerotic margin?

a. Osteogenic sarcoma
b. Ewing's sarcoma

c. Osteoid osteoma
d. Rickets

Answer c. Osteoid osteoma

Osteoid osteoma is characterized by a painful lesion in the second decade of life more commonly seen in men with radiographs that reveal a small round central lucency with a sclerotic margin. The treatment is nonsteroidal antiinflammatory drugs because the condition will resolve spontaneously.

> **Orders:**
> • *Naproxen*
>
> *Turn the clock forward, and the case will end.*

What is the most appropriate treatment for a patient with Ewing's sarcoma?

a. Chemotherapy
b. Radiation

c. Surgery
d. All of the above

Answer d. All of the above

The most appropriate therapy for a patient with Ewing's sarcoma is multidrug chemotherapy as well as local disease control with surgery and radiation.

> **Orders:**
> • *Hematology oncology consult*
> • *Surgery consult*
>
> *Turn the clock forward, and the case will end.*

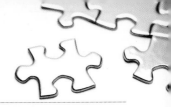

CHAPTER **9**

GASTROINTESTINAL

CASE 1: Pink Baby Sometimes

Setting: *Office*

CC: *"My baby is blue and then sometimes pink."*

Vitals: *Stable*

HPI: *A newborn child is brought for her first well-baby exam by a frantic mother. The mother states when the child is alone or feeding, she notices the baby is blue. On stimulation, the baby cries and then suddenly becomes pink. When an attempt to introduce a feeding catheter through the nose is made, there is considerable difficulty.*

PMH:
• *Holosystolic murmur*
• *The child does not startle with loud noises.*

What is the most likely diagnosis?

a. Choanal atresia

b. Esophageal atresia (EA)

c. Tracheoesophageal fistula (TEF)

d. Pyloric stenosis

Answer a. Choanal atresia

Choanal atresia is caused a failure in apoptosis, which leads to a membranous septum to remain between the nose and pharynx. This results in the child being unable to breathe through the nose and having subsequent cyanosis after trying to drink or eat. The child may have other symptoms of CHARGE syndrome, such as a holosystolic murmur indicative of ventricular septal defect. EA and TEF present with regurgitation and choking after feeding, and pyloric stenosis is characterized by projectile vomiting.

> C: Coloboma of the eye
> H: Heart defects
> A: Atresia of the choanae
> R: Retardation of development
> G: Genital defects
> E: Ear anomalies and deafness

The most accurate test for CHARGE syndrome involves specific genetic testing for the CHD7 gene.

CHD7 is a member of the chromodomain helicase DNA-binding (CHD) protein seen in patients with CHARGE.

What is the best initial test for test for diagnosing choanal atresia?

a. Nasogastric (NG) tube placement
b. Radiography of the neck
c. Fiberoptic rhinoscopy
d. Computed tomography (CT) scan of the head and neck

Answer a. Nasogastric (NG) tube placement

The best initial test is an unsuccessful attempt to pass an NG tube 3 to 4 cm into the nasopharynx. The most accurate test is to obtain a CT scan of the head and neck. Radiography of the neck will not reveal any excess tissues, and fiberoptic rhinoscopy is only used if the diagnosis is equivocal.

Orders:
• *Radiography*

Turn the clock forward, and the case scenario will state that the NG tube was unsuccessfully placed.

An NG tube cannot be placed.

The most common genital condition associated with CHARGE syndrome in boys is cryptorchidism.

What is the best treatment for this patient?

a. Surgical repair
b. Observation

Answer a. Surgical repair

Surgical repair is the correct answer for a patient who has choanal atresia. Typically, a transnasal repair is the most common approach and offers excellent outcomes.

Orders:

• *Surgical consult*

Turn the clock forward, and the case will end.

CASE 2: My Baby Dislikes Milk

Setting: *ED*

CC: *"My baby chokes every time he drinks milk."*

Vitals: *Stable*

HPI: *A 3-day-old premature boy is noted by his mother to choke. The mother reports that the child begins to suckle and then develops frothing, bubbling, and coughing with respiratory distress accompanied by cyanosis. She says that today when she tried to feed him again, he immediately began to regurgitate and aspirated.*

Physical Exam:
- *Radial aplasia of the right arm (Figure 9-1)*
- *Second to fourth rib deformities*
- *Holosystolic murmur*

What is the most likely diagnosis?

a. Duodenal atresia

b. Esophageal atresia (EA) with tracheoesophageal fistula (TEF)

c. Biliary atresia

d. Pyloric stenosis

Answer b. Esophageal atresia (EA) with tracheoesophageal fistula (TEF)

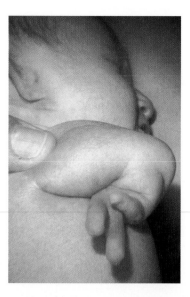

Figure 9-1. Radial aplasia of the right arm as seen in the VACTERL associations. (Reproduced with permission from CDC at http://phil.cdc.gov/phil_images/20021209/5/PHIL_2635_lores.jpg.)

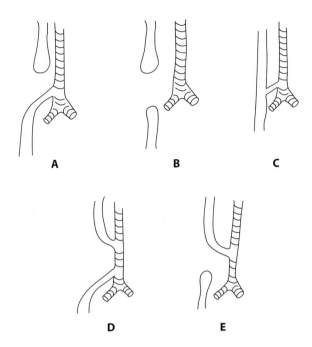

Figure 9-2. Types of esophageal atresia (EA) and tracheoesophageal fistula (TEF) **A,** Type 1, EA with distal TEF. **B,** Type 2, EA without TEF. **C,** Type 3, TEF without EA. **D,** Type 4, EA with proximal and distal TEF. **E,** Type 5, EA with proximal TEF. (Reproduced with permission from Gonzales KD, Lee H. Chapter 35. Congenital disorders of the trachea & esophagus. In: Lalwani AK, ed. *CURRENT Diagnosis & Treatment in Otolaryngology—Head & Neck Surgery.* 3rd ed. New York, NY: McGraw-Hill; 2012.)

Esophageal atresia (EA) is an abnormal connection or ending to the trachea and esophagus. There are five kinds of EA, with TEF as seen in Figure 9-2. The most common anatomic variant is the upper esophagus, which ends in a blind pouch and has a TEF. Patients present with regurgitation and aspiration after feeding. The most common type of EA is with TEF. A patient with duodenal atresia would present with bilious vomiting with every feeding. Biliary atresia presents with jaundice, hepatomegaly, and pale stools. Pyloric stenosis is characterized by projectile vomiting after feedings and a palpable mass in the abdomen.

EAs are associated with VACTERL malformations.
 V: Vertebral anomalies
 A: Anal atresia
 C: Cardiovascular anomalies
 TE: Tracheoesophageal fistula
 R: Renal (kidney) or radial anomalies (or both)
 L: Limb defects

> The most common cardiovascular malformation in the VACTERL malformations is a ventricular septal defect.

What is the best initial diagnostic test for a patient suspected to have EA?

a. Place an NG tube with radiography
b. Radiography

c. Esophagram
d. Upper endoscopy

Answer a. Place an NG tube with radiography

The inability to pass an NG tube aids in diagnosing EA. Radiography taken afterward may show a coiled NG tube in the blind pouch with no distal gas, also known as gasless abdomen. An esophagram with water-soluble contrast is used in patients with an isolated TEF. Upper endoscopy is typically not used unless there is a contraindication to contrast media.

> A fetus with EA cannot effectively swallow amniotic fluid, which in turn may lead to polyhydramnios, which in turn may lead to premature labor.

> Aspiration of saliva or milk can lead to an aspiration pneumonitis caused by lung exposure to gastric secretions.

Orders:
• *NG tube placement*
• *Radiography*

An NGT placed demonstrates coiling in the upper chest as seen in Figure 9-3.

> The most common anal malformation in the VACTERL malformations is imperforate anus.

What is the most appropriate therapy for this patient?

a. Percutaneous endoscopic gastrostomy
  (PEG) tube placement
b. Surgery

c. Observation
d. Endoscopic therapy

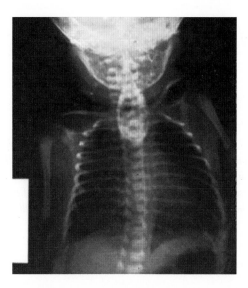

Figure 9-3. Esophageal atresia with tracheoesophageal fistula. Note the catheter coiled in the upper pouch. (Reproduced with permission from Hackam DJ, et al. Chapter 39. Pediatric surgery. In: Brunicardi F, et al., eds. *Schwartz's Principles of Surgery*. 9th ed. New York, NY: McGraw-Hill; 2010.)

Answer b. Surgery

Surgical ligation of the TEF with end-to-end anastomosis of the blind pouch esophagus to the stomach would be done. PEG tube placement is not indicated in this patient because surgical management is the best therapy. Observation alone is dangerous. The child will develop aspiration pneumonia. Endoscopic therapy cannot create the right anastomosis between the esophagus and stomach.

Orders:
• *Surgical consult*

Turn the clock forward, and the case will end.

Potter syndrome = bilateral renal agenesis = 100% mortality rate; therefore, surgical repair is contraindicated. Palliative care consult is the best next step in this case.

CASE 3: My Baby Vomits

Setting: *ED*

CC: *"My baby vomits after every meal."*

Vitals: *Stable except for tachycardia*

HPI: *A 5-week-old boy is presented with severe projectile vomiting after each meal that the mother describes as nonbilious in nature. The mother states the child has had such episodes since birth. He is still hungry and has a desire to feed more. The vomiting has become more intense, and at times the mother has noted bright red flecks. A baseline basic metabolic profile shows a hypochloremic, hypokalemic, metabolic alkalosis.*

ROS:
• *Flatus*
• *Loose bowel movements*

Physical Exam:
• *A small, firm, movable, olive-shaped mass is palpated in the mid-epigastrium. The mass is movable, and while the child is lying flat, a peristaltic wave can be seen.*

What is the most likely diagnosis?

a. Duodenal atresia
b. Pyloric stenosis
c. Gastroenteritis
d. Small bowel obstruction

Answer b. Pyloric stenosis

Pyloric stenosis is characterized by nonbilious, projectile vomiting after attempting to feed. The vomit lacks bile because of the inability of bile to reflux from the duodenum into the stomach. The child will still be hungry and have a desire to feed more, and because of the massive loss of hydrochloric acid, the child will have a hypochloremic, hypokalemic, metabolic alkalosis. Duodenal atresia presents with bilious vomiting. Gastroenteritis is caused by an infectious source and would not include a palpable mass in the abdomen. A small bowel obstruction can present with vomiting but would not have physical findings such as a palpable mass and would not have flatus and bowel movements, which this patient has.

What is the next best step in the management of this patient?

a. Correct the electrolytes
b. Ultrasonography
c. Intravenous (IV) fluids with normal saline
d. Endoscopy
e. Upper gastrointestinal (GI) series

Answer c. Intravenous (IV) fluids with normal saline

Before the establishment of the diagnosis, it is imperative that the patient's volume and electrolyte imbalances are corrected. The patient should be given IV normal saline to resuscitate his intravascular volume and then be given potassium repletion. The child should also be kept NPO (nothing by mouth) because that is the nidus for his vomiting. Ultrasonography is the best diagnostic test but should not be done before resuscitation. There is no role for endoscopy at this time in this patient. An upper GI series is less accurate than ultrasonography.

Gastric vomiting leads to the loss of hydrogen and chloride. This causes a hypochloremic metabolic acidosis and hypokalemia. The hypokalemia is caused by the secondary rise in aldosterone from hypovolemia, which causes the body to excrete potassium in place of sodium.

Volume contraction leads to increased levels of aldosterone. Increased aldosterone increases potassium and hydrogen excretion. Potassium and hydrogen ions are excreted at the late distal tubule.

Intercalated cells excrete hydrogen ions (acid).
Principal cells excrete potassium.

Pyloric stenosis is caused by hypertrophy and hyperplasia of the muscular layers of the pylorus, which leads to narrowing of the channel, which can easily lead to gastric outlet obstruction.

Orders:
- *IV access*
- *Normal saline*
- *IV potassium*
- *Ultrasonography of the abdomen*

Deregulation of vasoactive intestinal peptide (VIP) and nitric oxide is seen in the etiology of pyloric stenosis.

The child receives IV fluid with potassium repletion. Ultrasonography of the abdomen reveals a targetlike appearance, a pyloric wall thickness of 6 mm, and a pyloric channel length greater than 14 mm (Figure 9-4).

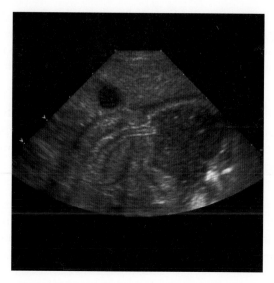

Figure 9-4. Ultrasound image showing pyloric stenosis. (Reproduced with permission from Niket Sonpal.)

Pyloric stenosis
- Target sign on ultrasonography
- String sign on upper GI series
- Railroad track sign on upper GI series

Pyloric wall thickness greater than 3 mm and pyloric channel length greater than 14 mm are abnormal.

What is the most appropriate therapy?

a. Endoscopic pylorotomy

b. Surgical pylorotomy

c. Medical therapy

d. Antiemetics

Answer b. Surgical pylorotomy

Surgical intervention is the most appropriate therapy for a patient with pyloric stenosis. Endoscopic balloon dilatation of pyloric stenosis is used after surgical therapy fails. There is no medical therapy that treats the underlying hypertrophy, and antiemetics are only needed if the child has persistent vomiting.

Prokinetic agents such as metoclopramide and erythromycin are contraindicated in children with pyloric stenosis as antiemetics.

Mechanism of action of metoclopramide
• Antiemetic D2 receptors antagonist
• Mixed 5-HT3–5-HT4 receptor antagonism
• Prokinetic activity D2 receptor antagonist with 5-HT4 receptor agonism

Orders:
• *Surgical consult*

Pyloric stenosis has no long-term impact on the child's future.

CASE 4: My Child Vomits All the Time

Setting: *ED*

CC: *"My child vomits green after every meal."*

Vitals: *Within normal limits except for tachycardia*

HPI: *A 1-day-old premature infant is presented with green bilious vomiting after each meal. The mother states that he is very irritable and constantly crying and hungry. She has attempted to feed him, but he vomits every time. The child was delivered after having polyhydramnios prenatally. Radiography done at the outpatient clinic showed two gas bubbles with no distal bowel gas (Figure 9-5).*

ROS:
• *No flatus*

Physical Exam:
• *Features of Down syndrome*
• *Soft and nondistended*

What is the most likely diagnosis?

a. Duodenal atresia

b. Pyloric stenosis

c. Gastroenteritis

d. Small bowel obstruction

Answer a. Duodenal atresia

Duodenal atresia presents with bilious vomiting without abdominal distension because the obstruction is just distal to the ampulla of Vater. Pyloric stenosis presents differently

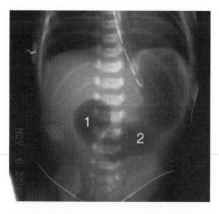

Figure 9-5. Abdominal radiograph showing the "double-bubble" sign in a newborn infant with duodenal atresia. The two bubbles are numbered. (Reproduced with permission from Hackam DJ, et al. Chapter 39. Pediatric surgery. In: Brunicardi F, et al., eds. *Schwartz's Principles of Surgery.* 9th ed. New York, NY: McGraw-Hill; 2010.)

because it has nonbilious vomiting. Small bowel obstruction present with vomiting and no flatus or bowel movements. However, radiographic findings would not have a double-bubble sign but rather multiple air-fluid levels. Gastroenteritis has a nonspecific gas pattern on radiographs.

> The duodenum develops from the caudal portion of the foregut and cranial portion of the midgut.

> Whereas duodenal atresia has no abdominal distension, jejunal and ileal atresia have significant abdominal distension.

What is the next best step in the management of this patient?

a. NG tube decompression
b. IV fluids
c. Electrolyte replacement
d. Antibiotics
e. Surgical duodenodenostomy
f. All of the above

Answer e. Surgical duodenodenostomy

The mainstay of therapy is surgical duodenodenostomy, but before surgery, it is important to place an NG tube, give the child IV fluids, and replace electrolytes. The commonly seen electrolyte abnormalities is hypokalemia, and the acid–base imbalance seen is a metabolic alkalosis.

> **Orders:**
> • *NGT tube placement*
> • *Chemistry (basic metabolic profile [BMP])*
> • *IV fluids*
> • *Electrolyte replacement*
> • *Surgical consult*
>
> *Turn the clock forward, and the case will end.*

> One third of patients with duodenal atresia have Down syndrome (trisomy 21).

CASE 5: Cystic Fibrosis

Setting: *ED*

CC: *"My child has not passed any stool."*

Vitals: *Stable*

HPI: *A 1-day-old infant has not passed meconium in the first 24 hours of life and has been vomiting. Her mother, who is very concerned, brings in the child to the emergency department. The child has been very irritable since birth and barely sleeps. Radiography completed 1 hour earlier shows a ground-glass or soap bubble appearance.*

ROS:
• *Multiple episodes of vomiting*

Physical Exam:
• *Abdominal distension*
• *Painful to palpation*
• *Normal rectal exam and tone*
• *Loops of bowel are palpable and feel cordlike*

What is the most likely diagnosis?

a. Duodenal atresia

b. Hirschsprung's disease

c. Malrotation

d. Meconium ileus

Answer d. Meconium ileus

The most likely diagnosis is meconium ileus. This is from the terminal ileum becoming obstructed by the thick meconium and is seen with neonates with cystic fibrosis (CF). In CF, the GI secretions are highly viscid and stick to the intestinal mucosa.

Hirschsprung's disease would have a gush of gas and stool on digital rectal exam, but this patient had a normal rectal exam. Malrotation would present bilious emesis and obstruction, but the plain film would show a gasless abdomen.

> Meconium consists of bile salts, bile acids, and debris that is shed from the intestinal mucosa.

> In meconium ileus, the obstruction occurs at the terminal ileum; in meconium plug syndrome, the obstruction is in the large bowel.

A "soap bubble" or "ground-glass" appearance caused by small air bubbles mixed with the meconium is diagnostic of meconium ileus.

What is the next best step in the management of this patient?

a. NPO

b. NG tube

c. IV fluids

d. Replace electrolytes

e. Water-soluble contrast enema

f. All of the above

Answer f. All of the above

The best initial therapy for a child with obstruction from meconium ileus is to make the child NPO, replace vascular volume, provide electrolytes with IV fluids, and decompress the bowel proximal to the terminal ileum. The most definitive therapy to give the child an enema with hypertonic water-soluble contrast, which will draw fluid into the bowel and cause the meconium to wash out.

There are no air-fluid levels in meconium ileus because the secretions are very thick and viscous and do not form layers.

Orders:
- *BMP*
- *NPO*
- *NG tube placement*
- *IV access*
- *Normal saline*
- *Replace electrolytes*
- *Contrast enema*

Turn the clock forward, and the case will end.

If the enema does not relieve the obstruction, laparotomy is required.

CASE 6: My Baby Doesn't Poop

Setting: *Office*

CC: *"My baby doesn't poop very often."*

Vitals: *Stable*

HPI: *A newborn baby is brought in for an exam, and the mother complains that the baby has not pooped since his birth. His diapers have been clean except for urine. The mother is concerned because the child is irritable, and she thinks his belly is very distended. Her older brother had a similar problem when he was a baby and needed surgery.*

Physical Exam:
• *Severe abdominal distension is noted.*
• *Upon rectal exam with a pinky, a large release of stool and gas is noted.*

What is the most likely diagnosis?

a. Malrotation

b. Volvulus

c. Hirschsprung's disease

d. Imperforate anus

e. Intussusception

Answer c. Hirschsprung's disease

Hirschsprung's disease is the congenital absence of the ganglionic cells in the submucosal and myenteric plexus. This leads to excessive smooth muscle tone at the rectum, leading to uncoordinated peristalsis and contractility. Whereas malrotation is caused by incomplete rotation of the intestine during fetal development, volvulus is more common in a setting of previous bowel surgery with a history of bilious emesis. Imperforate anus presents with distension, but the child lacks an actual orifice of the release of stool. Intussusception is the telescoping of bowel presenting with currant jelly stool.

Three nerve plexi innervate the intestine: the submucosal (Meissner) plexus, the myenteric (Auerbach) plexus, and the smaller mucosal plexus.

The underlying problem is an arrest of neuroblasts from migrating and descending into the proximal distal large bowel.

The most common cause of intestinal obstruction in a neonate is Hirschsprung's disease.

What is the next best step in the management of this patient?

a. Radiography of the abdomen

b. Barium enema

c. Rectal biopsy

d. Anorectal manometry

Answer b. Barium enema

The best initial test is a barium enema, which will help demonstrate a narrow distal colon with proximal dilation. Radiography of the abdomen will show distended bowel loops but is very nonspecific, and the most accurate test is a suction rectal biopsy. The biopsy would show a lack of ganglionic cells. Anorectal manometry can be used to correlate the findings but does not have greater sensitivity and specificity than a biopsy.

Orders:

• *Barium enema*

• *GI consult*

• *Colonoscopy with biopsy*

Turn the clock forward to obtain biopsy results. The patient may need to be sent home and brought back to the office.

A barium enema is performed, which demonstrates a narrow distal colon. A colonoscopy with biopsy is performed. Pathologic analysis shows a lack of ganglionic cells.

What is the most appropriate therapy for a patient with Hirschsprung's disease?

a. Stool softeners

b. Prokinetic agents

c. Surgical therapy

d. Endoscopic rectal stenting

Answer c. Surgical therapy

Treatment of patients with Hirschsprung's disease consists of laparoscopic removal of the abnormal section of the colon followed by reanastomosis. Stool softeners and prokinetic agents have not been shown to be helpful, and endoscopic rectal stenting is only used as a palliative procedure in rectal adenocarcinoma.

CASE 7: Bloody Diarrhea

Setting: *ED*

CC: *"My baby has had blood in his diaper."*

Vitals: *Stable*

HPI: *A 2-year-old boy is presented with 2 weeks of blood in his diaper that is noted in his stool. The baby does not cry when he passes stool. The mother describes his stools as currant jelly.*

ROS:
- *No nausea*
- *No vomiting*
- *No diarrhea*

Physical Exam:
- *Soft, nontender abdomen with a palpable mass in the mid-abdomen*
- *Rectal examination is normal*
- *Stool in the diaper is dark red consistent with hematochezia*

What is the most likely diagnosis?

a. Meckel's diverticulum

b. Intussusception

c. Peptic ulcer disease

d. Necrotizing enterocolitis

Answer a. Meckel's diverticulum

Meckel's diverticulum is the most common cause of painless bleeding in an infant. It is caused by gastric acid–secreting mucosa that is ectopic to the intestine that causes bleeding by searing the mucosa of the small bowel. Intussusception would present with currant jelly stools but would have painful episodes of crampy abdominal pain, and peptic ulcer disease would present with melena and epigastric pain. Necrotizing enterocolitis is seen in premature newborns and is characterized by gas in the bowel wall and sepsis.

Meckel's diverticulum is the most common congenital abnormality of the small intestine.

It is caused by an incomplete obliteration of the omphalomesenteric duct.

Meckel's diverticulum is a true diverticulum that contains all of the layers normally found in the ileum.

Hematochezia is the most common presenting sign followed by obstruction and diverticulitis.

What is the best diagnostic test for this patient?

a. Colonoscopy

b. Upper endoscopy

c. Technetium-99m scintiscan

d. Small bowel capsule study

Answer c. Technetium-99m scintiscan

The best diagnostic test for a patient suspected to have Meckel's diverticulum is a technetium-99m scintiscan, also known as a Meckel's scan. The technetium-99m is taken up by heterotopic gastric mucosa and therefore on scanning localizes the site of a Meckel's diverticulum. Upper endoscopy, colonoscopy, and small bowel capsule are used in the evaluation of bleeding but are not the best tests in the evaluation of Meckel's diverticulum. Meckel's diverticulum is located in the small bowel, which is by definition hard to reach by endoscopy. Lower endoscopy reaches to the ileocecal valve, and Meckel's diverticulum is located more proximal than that.

There are two types of mucosa in Meckel diverticulum, gastric and intestinal.

Orders:
- *Complete blood count (CBC)*
- *Meckel's scan*

A abdominal Technetium-99m (Tc-99m) pertechnetate scintigraphy was performed and shows uptake above the diverticulum as seen in Figure 9-6. CBC shows hemoglobin of 12.1 g/dL.

What is the most appropriate therapy for a patient with Meckel's diverticulum?

a. Endoscopic resection

b. Proton pump inhibitors (PPIs)

c. Surgical excision

d. H2 blockers

Answer c. Surgical excision

Surgical excision of the diverticulum is the most appropriate therapy for a patient who presents with symptomatic ectopic gastric tissue. Endoscopic resection is not possible because it is difficult to localize from within the lumen. PPI therapy and H2 blockers will only suppress gastric acid release but will not treat the underlying cause of bleeding.

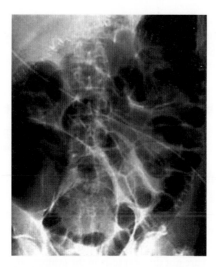

Figure 9-6. This abdominal technetium-99m pertechnetate scintigraphy was performed 15 minutes after the radionuclide injection. The spherical area of increased uptake *(arrow)* a few centimeters above the bladder corresponds to a Meckel diverticulum. This diagnosis was confirmed by surgery. (Reproduced with permission from McQuaid KR. Chapter 15. Gastrointestinal disorders. In: Papadakis MA, McPhee SJ, Rabow MW, eds. *CURRENT Medical Diagnosis & Treatment 2014.* New York, NY: McGraw-Hill; 2014.)

Orders:
• *Surgical consult*
• *After surgery, admit the patient to the intensive care unit.*

Turn the clock forward, and the case will end.

Rule of 2s for Meckel's diverticulum
• 2% of population
• 2% symptomatic
• 2 inches long
• 2 feet from ileocecal valve
• 2 types of tissue

CASE 8: Currant Jelly Again

Setting: *ED*

CC: *"My baby has currant jelly in his diaper."*

Vitals: *Within normal limits except for a fever of 100.9°F and tachycardia*

HPI: *An 18-month-old boy is seen for abdominal pain that has lasted for 3 days. The most recent episodes were associated with bilious vomiting and fever. The mother states he has had currant jelly in his diaper for the last three bowel movements. She is unaware of who keeps feeding her child currant jelly and thinks it's his older brother. The mother notes that when the child is in pain, he brings his knees up to his chest.*

PMH:
- *Otitis media 1 week ago*

Physical Exam:
- *Sausage-shaped mass and emptiness in the right lower quadrant*
- *Distended abdomen*
- *Rectal exam is normal*
- *No peritoneal signs*

What is the most likely diagnosis?

a. *Clostridium difficile* infection
b. Intussusception
c. Meckel's diverticulum
d. Peptic ulcer disease
e. Anal fissure

Answer b. Intussusception

Intussusception is when the bowel telescopes into itself, leading to colicky pain with the legs flexed at peak pain, bloody stools that appear like currant jelly, and vomiting. Patients may also have fevers, lethargy, and a sausage-shaped mass in the right lower colon. *C. difficile* infection presents with nonbloody diarrhea after exposure to antibiotics, and Meckel diverticulum would have currant jelly stools but would not have a mass on the right lower quadrant. A patient with peptic ulcer disease would have melena and epigastric pain. Patients with anal fissure have pain only on passing stools, and it would be bright red in nature.

Bowel telescoping causes arterial and venous obstruction and mucous necrosis, which when combined, leads to the classical currant jelly stools.

The most common place for intussusception is at the ileal-colic region.

What is the next best diagnostic step in the management of this patient?

a. Ultrasonography

b. Air enema

c. Barium enema

d. Radiography of the abdomen

e. CBC

Answer a. Ultrasonography

Ultrasonography is the best initial test for patient suspected of having intussusception; the findings most associated with the findings are a "doughnut sign." An air enema is the most accurate study of choice because it is both diagnostic and therapeutic in nature. A barium enema is not indicated because there is a chance of perforation. Barium leaking into the abdominal cavity is caustic to the peritoneum. A CBC should be checked routinely in all patients who are bleeding but does not offer much in the way of diagnostic information for this patient.

Intussusception is associated with adenovirus and episodes of otitis media.

Rotavirus is a double-stranded RNA virus and is transmitted by the fecal oral route.

Leading points can also cause intussusception, including a Meckel's diverticulum, polyp, neurofibroma, and malignancy.

Leading points are
• Lesion or variation in the intestine
• Trapped by peristalsis
• Dragged into distal segment of intestine

Orders:
• CBC
• Ultrasound
• Air enema

Ultrasonography of the abdomen reveals a doughnut appearance and no free air, as seen in Figure 9-7. An air enema is performed without any complications. A CBC shows hemoglobin of 13.1 g/dL. The child's fever has normalized. The patient has not cried and appears much more comfortable.

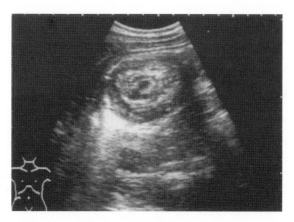

Figure 9-7. Ultrasound image of intussusception showing the classic target appearance of bowel within bowel. (Reproduced with permission from Kharbanda AB, Sawaya RD. Chapter 124. Acute abdominal pain in children. In: Tintinalli JE, et al., eds. *Tintinalli's Emergency Medicine: A Comprehensive Study Guide.* 7th ed. New York, NY: McGraw-Hill; 2011.)

Orders:
- *If the child feels better, turn the clock forward, and the case will end.*
- *If the case does not end or free air is seen, order a surgical consult and admit the child postoperatively*

If the patient has peritoneal signs or perforation (free air) or presents with shock, surgery is the best therapy, and air enema will not help.

Air enema physically pushes the bowel back into place. This is successful in 90% of patients.

CASE 9: My Kid Has a Rash on His Bottom

Setting: *ED*

CC: *"My kid has a rash on his bottom."*

Vitals: *Stable*

HPI: *An 8-year-old boy is brought to the emergency department by his father with a rash on his lower extremities and buttocks, abdominal pain, and joint pain. The child says the rash is itchy; he has vomited twice. The pain in his joints has been mostly localized to his knees and ankles. The father states the child recently had an upper respiratory infection. CBC reveals thrombocytosis; coagulation profiles and electrolytes are within normal limits.*

ROS:
- *Cola-colored urine*
- *Swollen joints*

PE:
- *Knees are warm and swollen bilaterally*
- *Maculopapular blanching rash below the waist; in certain areas, petechiae and purpura are seen (Figure 9-8)*
- *No peripheral edema*

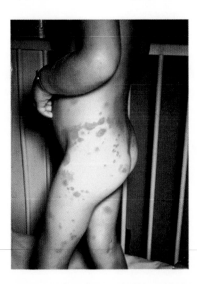

Figure 9-8. Henoch-Schönlein purpura (HSP). This child has palpable purpura on the extensor surfaces of the legs. HSP should be considered whenever there is symmetric ecchymosis along the extensor surfaces of the extremities and buttocks. Migratory arthritis and abdominal pain may be present. (Reproduced with permission from Shapiro RA, et al. Chapter 15. Child abuse. In: Knoop KJ, Stack LB, Storrow AB, Thurman R, eds. *The Atlas of Emergency Medicine.* 3rd ed. New York, NY: McGraw-Hill; 2010.)

What is the most likely diagnosis?

a. DIC

b. Henoch-Schonlein purpura (HSP)

c. Renal failure

d. Immune thrombocytopenia (ITP)

e. Thrombotic thrombocytopenic purpura (TTP)

Answer b. Henoch-Schonlein purpura (HSP)

HSP presents at the classic triad of abdominal pain, arthralgias, and purpura. HSP is an IgA-mediated vasculitis of the small vessel. Disseminated intravascular coagulation is not possible because the patient has normal coagulation profiles, and TTP would present with fever, anemia, thrombocytopenia, renal failure, and neurologic dysfunction. Renal failure alone is not the diagnosis, but patients with HSP can have impaired renal function glomerulonephritis. ITP is an autoimmune thrombocytopenia, which is a diagnosis of exclusion but cannot be valid here because the patient has normal platelets.

> HSP is caused by complexes of immunoglobulin A (IgA) and complement component 3 (C3) being deposited into arterioles, capillaries, and venules.

> Purpura + High platelets = HSP
> Purpura + Low platelets = TTP, ITP, or other low platelet conditions.

> The joints most commonly affected in HSP are the knees and ankles.

What is the diagnostic test of choice in this patient?

a. Clinical diagnosis

b. Skin biopsy

c. Renal biopsy

d. IgA level

e. Response to steroids

Answer a. Clinical diagnosis

The diagnosis of HSP is made through clinical diagnosis; a definitive diagnosis is made through skin biopsy of one of these purpuric lesions. A renal biopsy will show mesangial deposition of IgA, but that is nonspecific because there are other IgA nephropathies.

> IgA and IGM are elevated in patients with HSP.

> Factor XIII is reduced in about 50% of patients with HSP.

What is the best therapy for this patient?

a. Symptomatic treatment

b. Corticosteroids

c. Intravenous immunoglobulin (IVIG)

d. Nonsteroidal antiinflammatory drugs (NSAIDs)

Answer a. Symptomatic treatment

Symptomatic treatment is the best therapy because this patient's disease is self-limited. However, steroids should be used if the patient has intestinal complications such as GI bleeds or persistent renal impairment. IVIG is used in patients with refractory disease or brain bleeds, and NSAIDs are used for the symptomatic control of joint pain.

Answer steroids for the following:
• Persistent nephrotic syndrome
• Severe tissue edema
• GI hemorrhage
• Scrotal edema

Orders:
• *Ibuprofen*
• *Send the patient home and bring him back in 2 weeks.*

Turn the clock forward, and the patient will improve.

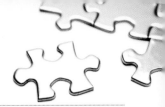

CHAPTER **10**

CARDIOLOGY

CASE 1: **Machines and Much More**

Setting: *NICU*

CC: *"I was just born."*

Vitals: *Within normal limits except for tachypnea*

HPI: *A newborn girl is 3 weeks old. Her mother had no prenatal care and developed a rubella infection during her gestation. On examination, the child is found to have difficulty with feeding.*

ROS:
- *Diaphoresis*
- *Low weight*

Physical Exam:
- *Tachypnea*
- *Apical impulse is laterally displaced with a thrill*
- *Normal S_1 with an obscured S_2 with a machinery murmur*
- *Peripheral pulses are bounding*

What is the most likely diagnosis?

a. Aortic stenosis

b. Patent ductus arteriosus (PDA)

c. Aortic regurgitation (AR)

d. Mitral regurgitation

e. Hypertrophic obstructive cardiomyopathy (HOCM)

Answer b. Patent ductus arteriosus (PDA)

PDA presents with a normal S_1 and an obscured S_2 with a machinery murmur. It is caused by the continued communication between the thoracic aorta and pulmonary artery, likely secondary to this patient's maternal rubella infection. Aortic stenosis presents with an early systolic ejection click at the upper right sternal border that radiates to the neck. AR is associated with bounding pulses and a wide pulse pressure, which are not seen in this patient. Mitral regurgitation presents with a holosystolic murmur that radiates to the axilla.

Ductus arteriosus is a persistent communication between the descending thoracic aorta and the pulmonary artery.

Peripheral pulses are often referred to as bounding. This is related to the high left ventricular stroke volume, which may cause systolic hypertension.

What is the next best step in the management of this patient?

a. Electrocardiography (ECG)

c. Chest radiography

b. Echocardiography

d. Observation and discharge

Answer b. Echocardiography

Echocardiography is the best initial diagnostic test in a patient with PDA. Echocardiography with Doppler imaging would show patent flow through the ductus arteriosus. An ECG would only show left ventricular hypertrophy (LVH), but this is not specific. A chest radiography would show nonspecific findings such increased pulmonary markings and cardiomegaly if congestive heart failure (CHF) has developed.

The ductus arteriosus is a remnant of the distal sixth aortic arch.

- Prostaglandin E2 pops open the ductus arteriosus.
- Increased PO_2, endothelin-1, norepinephrine, and acetylcholine close the ductus arteriosus.
- Nonsteroidal antiinflammatory drugs antagonize prostaglandins and close the ductus arteriosus.

Congenital rubella prevents closure of ductus arteriosus.

Orders:

• *Echocardiography*

An echocardiogram is performed and shows increased duct flow during diastole consistent with PDA.

What is the next best step in management?

a. Observation

c. Surgical closure

b. Indomethacin

Answer a. Observation

Most PDAs close spontaneously, and it is acceptable to observe the patient while she is asymptomatic and reevaluate in 6 to 12 months. However, patients who are premature or presenting with findings of CHF can be considered for closure with indomethacin or aspirin. If medical therapy is ineffective, patients are referred for surgical closure.

If the child is preterm and has a PDA, you must administer indomethacin as the next best step in management. Therapy is continued until B-type natriuretic peptide values decrease.

Brain natriuretic peptide is released by the cardiomyocytes in response to excessive stretching of heart muscle cells.

Unrepaired PDA is an indication for antibiotic prophylaxis during dental procedures.

CASE 2: Tetralogy of What?

Setting: *Office*

CC: *"My baby doesn't like to play."*

Vitals: *Stable*

HPI: *An 18-month-old girl presents with her mother, who says the girl is restless and irritable. She has difficulty with feeding and has episodes of turning blue and gasping for breath. The mother has noticed the child feels better when she squats.*

Physical Exam:
- *Smaller than expected for age*
- *Cyanosis of the lips and nail beds*
- *Clubbing of the fingernails*
- *Harsh systolic ejection murmur*

What is the most likely diagnosis?

a. HOCM

b. Coarctation of the aorta

c. Tetralogy of Fallot (TOF)

d. Ebstein's anomaly

Answer c. Tetralogy of Fallot (TOF)

TOF is a congenital heart defect characterized by an overriding aorta, pulmonary stenosis, ventricular septal defect (VSD), and right ventricular hypertrophy. This condition results in low oxygen content in the blood caused by the mixing of oxygenated blood through the VSD. The baby is cyanotic, and when she develops breathlessness, she will squat down to achieve increased oxygenation. The squatting causes increased peripheral vascular resistance and allows for a temporary reversal of the shunt. This causes more blood to flow into the lungs and a temporary rise in central oxygenation. A coarctation of the aorta is characterized by differential blood pressures between the upper and lower extremities.

HOCM is characterized by an overgrown septum, leading to ventricular outflow obstruction characterized by dyspnea, chest pain, and syncope. Ebstein's anomaly is seen in children of mothers who took lithium during gestation. Ebstein's anomaly is a tricuspid valve that is driven down into the right ventricle. It is ventricularization of the tricuspid valve.

TOF has four findings = four mutations
- *JAG1*
- *NKX2-5*
- *ZFPM2*
- *VEGF*

TOF + Patent foramen ovale or atrial septal defect = Pentalogy of Fallot

What is the best initial test for this patient?

a. Radiography of the chest

b. Magnetic resonance imaging (MRI) of the chest

c. Echocardiography

d. Angiography

Answer a. Chest radiography

Radiography of the chest shows a bootlike appearance of the heart with TOF. An MRI of the chest will offer greater anatomic delineation but is the not the best initial test. Echocardiography will usually reveal a large VSD with an overriding aorta and variable degrees of right ventricular outflow tract (RVOT) obstruction. Angiography is overly invasive at this time and is usually done electively before surgical repair.

Factors associated with a higher incidence of TOF include maternal rubella, poor prenatal nutrition, maternal alcohol use, and maternal age older than 40 years.

Untreated TOF can lead to paradoxical emboli that lead to strokes and pulmonary embolus.

Orders:
- *Chest radiography*
- *Echocardiogram*

Chest radiography reveals a boot-shaped heart (Figure 10-1), and echocardiography reveals a large VSD with an overriding aorta (Figure 10-2), and variable degrees of RVOT.

Prolonged cyanosis causes reactive polycythemia in order to increase oxygen-carrying capacity.

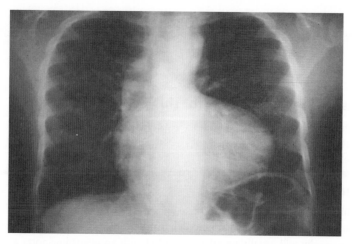

Figure 10-1. Chest radiograph revealing the classic "boot-shaped heart" of tetralogy of Fallot. (Reproduced with permission from Yee LL, Meckler GD. Chapter 122A. Pediatric heart disease: congenital heart defects. In: Tintinalli JE, et al., eds. *Tintinalli's Emergency Medicine: A Comprehensive Study Guide.* 7th ed. New York, NY: McGraw-Hill; 2011.)

> Automatic implantable cardiac defibrillator (AICD) placement is recommended in patients with TOF who develop sustained ventricular tachycardia or a sudden death event.

What is the most definitive therapy for this patient?

a. Surgical repair

b. Medical therapy

c. Palliative care

d. Continued imaging and observation

Answer a. Surgical repair

Surgical repair is the definitive therapy and is designed to reduce the right outflow obstruction. Palliative surgery is carried out by forming a side-to-end anastomosis between the subclavian artery. The pulmonary artery and is only reserved in patient's with concomitant pulmonary atresia and hypoplasia of the pulmonary artery. Medical therapy includes beta-blockers but is not the definitive therapy. Continued imaging and observation are incorrect and may lead to untoward effects.

> Survival is approximately 75% after the first year of life, 60% by 4 years, 30% by 10 years, and 5% by 40 years.

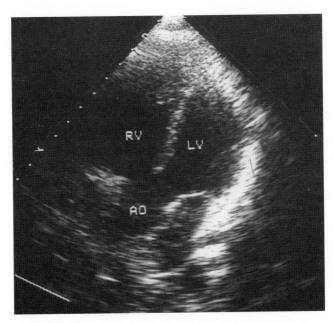

Figure 10-2. Images of tetralogy showing a large ventricular septal defect (VS) and overriding aorta (AO). LV, left ventricle; RV, right ventricle. (Reproduced with permission from DeMaria AN, Blanchard DG. Chapter 18. Echocardiography. In: Fuster V, Walsh RA, Harrington RA, eds. *Hurst's The Heart.* 13th ed. New York, NY: McGraw-Hill; 2011.)

Surgery for TOF must be completed by age 2.

Orders:
- *Cardiology consult*
- *Preoperative labs including complete blood count (CBC), complete metabolic profile (CMP), and coagulation profile*
- *Surgical consult*

Turn the clock forward, and the case will end.

CASE 3: Who is Ebstein?

Setting: *ED*

CC: *"My baby is blue."*

Vitals: *Stable except for tachypnea*

HPI: *A mother with bipolar disorder brings her 6-month-old child to the family practice clinic. The child is cyanotic on presentation. The mother states that the baby has been very listless and not as playful.*

Physical Exam:
- *Widely split first heart sound with loud tricuspid component*
- *S3 heart sound*
- *S4 heart sound*
- *Holosystolic murmur increased by inspiration*
- *2+ Peripheral edema*

What is the most likely diagnosis?

a. HOCM

b. Coarctation of the aorta

c. TOF

d. Ebstein's anomaly

Answer d. Ebstein's anomaly

Ebstein's anatomy is the development of a downward displaced tricuspid valve into the right ventricle lithium exposure to the fetus in utero. Over time, this will lead to atrialization of the right ventricle and malformation of the leaflets. The right atrium is dilated, and there will be a holosystolic murmur secondary to tricuspid regurgitation. It is usually accompanied by an atrial septal defect or patent foramen ovale.

The atrialized right ventricle gets split into parts, the very large atrialized component and the smaller small normal ventricle.

A delta wave is seen in a person with Wolff-Parkinson-White (WPW) syndrome.

Lithium exposure is a risk factor for the development of Ebstein's anomaly.

What is the next best step in the management of this patient?

a. Chest radiography

b. Echocardiography

c. ECG

d. Discharge home and follow up in 6 months

Answer a. Chest radiography

The best initial test for a child who presents with Ebstein's anomaly is to obtain an echocardiogram. Echocardiography is the most accurate test for many congenital cardiac lesions. Chest radiographs are not very useful for delineating an exact cause of cyanosis and are sensitive but not specific. This means that chest radiography findings are frequently abnormal but cannot show anything specific about the cardiac interior. ECG will show a tall QRS and broad P waves and a normal or prolonged PR interval.

Ebstein's anomaly is commonly associated with WPW syndrome.

Orders:

• *Echocardiography*

An echocardiogram demonstrates apical displacement of the septal leaflet of the tricuspid valve as seen in Figure 10-3.

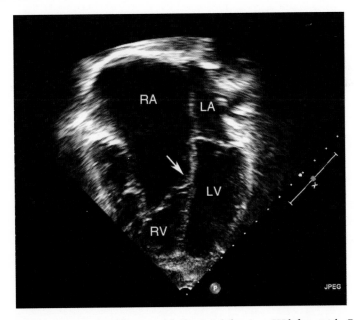

Figure 10-3. Ebstein's anomaly of the tricuspid valve. LA, left atrium; LV, left ventricle; RA, right atrium; RV, right ventricle. *Arrow* indicates. (Reproduced with permission from Brown DW, Fulton DR. Chapter 83. Congenital heart disease in children and adolescents. In: Fuster V, Walsh RA, Harrington RA, eds. *Hurst's The Heart*. 13th ed. New York, NY: McGraw-Hill; 2011.)

What is the best therapy for this patient?

a. Radiofrequency ablation (RFA)   **d.** All of the above
b. Surgery
c. Angiotensin-converting enzyme
   (ACE) inhibitors

Answer d. All of the above

RFA followed by surgery is done if the patient presents with WPW or supraventricular tachycardia. ACE inhibitors are used to slow the progression of the development of heart failure before surgery.

> **Orders:**
> • Cardiology consultation
> • Preoperative labs, including CBC, CMP, and coagulation profile
> • Surgical consult
>
> Turn the clock forward, and the case will end.

CASE 4: Transposition

Setting: *Office*

CC: *"My newborn is cyanotic."*

Vitals: *Stable except for tachypnea*

HPI: *A less than 1-day-old boy who was born at term is cyanotic and short of breath. The cyanosis developed within the past 6 hours.*

Physical Exam:
- *Severe cyanosis*
- *Single loud S$_2$*
- *Holosystolic murmur at the lower sternal border*

What is the most likely diagnosis?

a. Transposition of the great arteries (TGA)

b. Coarctation of the aorta

c. Truncus arteriosus

d. Total anomalous pulmonary venous return (TAPVR)

Answer a. Transposition of the great arteries (TGA)

TGA is a cyanotic condition in which the aorta arises from the right ventricle. The exact causes and etiology of the condition are unknown, but it presents with cyanosis unless there are a patent PDA and foramen ovale. Coarctation of the aorta presents with differential blood pressures from upper and lower extremities. TAPVR is the incorrect drainage of pulmonary veins into systemic venous circulation.

There is abnormal persistence of the subaortic conus with abnormal development of the subpulmonary conus. This causes the aorta to misalign with the right ventricle during development, leading to abnormal blood flow and cyanosis.

TAPVR and TGA are both cyanotic lesions. The main difference is that in TGA, the aorta stems from the right ventricle, providing no oxygenated blood to the body. TAPVR causes the pulmonary veins to drain into the systemic venous return, causing cyanosis.

What is the next best step in the management of this patient?

a. Chest radiography

b. Echocardiography

c. ECG

d. Angiography

Answer b. Echocardiography

Echocardiography is the next best step in the diagnosis of TGA. It will demonstrate aortic flow stemming from the right ventricle and abnormalities of the coronary vessels as well. Chest radiography is the best initial test and will show an "egg-on-string" appearance. This is attributable to a narrow heart base plus absence of the pulmonary artery's main segment.

> VSD leads to cardiomegaly and increased pulmonary vascular markings because of increased blood flow.

> TGA is the most common cyanotic lesion presenting in the immediate newborn period.

Orders:
- *Chest radiography*
- *Echocardiography*

Chest radiography reveals an eggs-on-string appearance, and echocardiography reveals a VSD, patent PDA, atrial septum, cardiomegaly, and Doppler aortic flow stemming from the right ventricle.

What is the next best step in the management of this patient?

a. Prostaglandin E1 (PGE1) therapy

b. Arterial switch therapy

c. Both a and b

d. No therapy needed

Answer c. Both a and b

The therapy for TGA involves medical therapy with infusion of PGE1 to maintain the opening of the PDA to allow for blood to flow into the systemic circulation while the child is prepared to have an arterial switch therapy.

> TGA is more commonly seen in the infants of mothers with diabetes.

Orders:
- Cardiology consultation
- Preoperative labs, including CBC, CMP, and coagulation profile
- Surgical consult

Turn the clock forward, and the case will end.

CASE 5: Single Truncus

Setting: *ED*

CC: *"My baby is blue."*

Vitals: *Stable*

HPI: *A 2-week-old newborn is progressively becoming more cyanotic. The mother is highly concerned and states that she had normal prenatal care. Chest radiography shows cardiomegaly, an ECG reveals large QRS complexes, and chest radiography shows an enlarged heart shadow with increased pulmonary blood flow. An echocardiogram shows a single outflow from the ventricles.*

Physical Exam:
- *Wide pulse pressure*
- *Cyanosis*
- *High-pitched early diastolic decrescendo at mid-left sternal border*
- *Single S$_2$*
- *Apical mid-diastolic rumble*
- *Crackles and rales*

What is the most likely diagnosis?

a. TGA

b. Coarctation of the aorta

c. Truncus arteriosus

d. TAPVR

Answer c. Truncus arteriosus

Truncus arteriosus (Figure 10-4) is the most likely condition when an infant presents with worsening cyanosis and findings of CHF. The condition is caused by a single arterial trunk arising from the ventricles by means of a single semilunar valve. The classic findings on exam include a single S$_2$ sound with a loud thrill, with minimal cyanosis. As the pulmonary vascular resistance decreases over time, more blood will flow into the pulmonary true, leading to bounding pulses and a widened pulse pressure.

Incomplete or failed septation of the embryonic truncus arteriosus leads to a persistence of the truncus arteriosus.

The most common associated finding with truncus arteriosus is regurgitating valves between the truncus and the two ventricles.

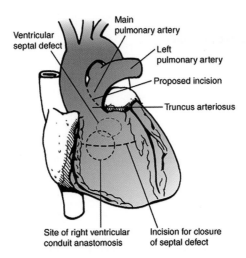

Ventricular septal defect

Main pulmonary artery

Left pulmonary artery

Proposed incision

Truncus arteriosus

Site of right ventricular conduit anastomosis

Incision for closure of septal defect

The main pulmonary artery arises from the truncus arteriosus downstream to the ... oduced with permission from Hirsh JC, et al. Chapter 19B. The heart: II. ... sease. In: Doherty GM, ed. *CURRENT Diagnosis & Treatment: Surgery*. 13th ed. ... Graw-Hill; 2010.)

next best step in the management of this patient?

c. Surgical repair
d. All of the above

Answer d. All of the above

The mainstay of treatment for a child with truncus arteriosus is to treat the heart failure with inotropic agents, diuretics, and complete surgical repair in the first few weeks of life.

Ductus arteriosus is derived from the sixth branchial arch.

Aortic arch is derived from the fourth branchial arch.

Babies with truncus arteriosus frequently present in shock because of high-output heart failure.

Orders:
- Cardiology consultation
- Preoperative labs, including CBC, CMP, and coagulation profile
- Surgical consult

Turn the clock forward, and the case will end.

CASE 6: Coarctation

Setting: *Office*

CC: *"I can't catch my breath."*

Vitals: *Stable*

HPI: *A 16-year-old male basketball player presents with shortness of breath that he experiences while at his practice games. He felt lightheaded the past few days but currently has no symptoms.*

Physical Exam:
- *Bifid pulse*
- *S_4 heart sound*
- *3/6 systolic murmurs at left sternal border that improves with hand grip and worsens with standing*
- *Apical precordial impulse that is displaced laterally*

An S_4 gallop is a sign of a noncompliant stiff left ventricle.

What is the most likely diagnosis?

a. HOCM

b. Aortic stenosis

c. AR

d. Coarctation of the aorta

Answer a. HOCM

HOCM is the most likely diagnosis for shortness of breath and near syncope in a male athlete. The murmur of HOCM is improved with handgrip and worsens with decreased preload. Aortic stenosis presents with a crescendo–decrescendo murmur, and AR would present with De Musset's sign and a diastolic murmur. De Musset's sign is head bobbing in timing with the cardiac cycle. This is because of the massive increase in stroke volume in AR. Coarctation of the aorta presents with differential blood pressures between the upper and lower extremities.

HOCM is an autosomal dominant trait.

Dyspnea is the most common presenting symptom of HOCM.

Sudden cardiac death is the most tragic presenting manifestation of HOCM.

What is the next best step in the management of this patient?

a. ECG

b. Chest radiography

c. Echocardiography

d. Multigated acquisition (MUGA) scan

Answer c. Echocardiography

Echocardiography is the next best step in the management of any patient who presents with signs and symptoms associated with HOCM. An ECG and chest radiography are sensitive for HOCM and will show left ventricular hypertrophy and cardiomegaly, respectively. A MUGA scan is the most accurate test to test of ejection fraction but is not needed for the diagnosis of HOCM.

Orders:

- *Cardiology consultation*
- *ECG*
- *Chest radiography*
- *Echocardiogram*

Chest radiography reveals cardiomegaly. ECG reveals ST-T wave abnormalities and LVH on echocardiography. Echocardiography reveals enlargement of the septum with left ventricular outflow impairment (Figure 10-5).

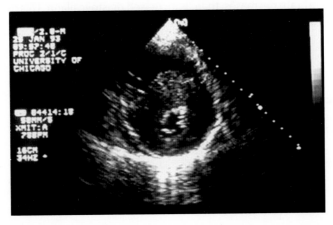

Figure 10-5. Hypertrophic cardiomyopathy. Short-axis two-dimensional echocardiographic view showing the left ventricle in cross-section. (Reproduced with permission from Sorrentino MJ. Chapter 29. Valvular heart disease. In: Hall JB, Schmidt GA, Wood LH, eds. *Principles of Critical Care.* 3rd ed. New York, NY: McGraw-Hill; 2005.)

Mutations occur in the β-myosin heavy chain gene on chromosome 14.

The most common ECG finding in HOCM non-specific ST changes.

What is the next best step in the management of this patient?

a. Start beta-blockers
b. No strenuous exercise or activity
c. Implantable cardioverter defibrillator (ICD)
d. Surgical myomectomy
e. All of the above

Answer d. Surgical myomectomy

The best initial therapy is to start beta-blockers and avoid exercise. Patients who have a high risk of sudden cardiac death should have an ICD placed. If the patient continues to experience symptoms or has unstable hemodynamics, he should then undergo surgical myomectomy. If surgical myomectomy is not an option, an alternative less invasive choice is catheter septal ablation.

Diuretics severely worsen symptoms of HOCM because of decreased preload.

Beta-blockers are effective because of their negative chronotropic effects. As the heart rate decreases, there is increased diastolic filling. This decreases the degree of obstruction on outflow through an increase of cardiac output.

Orders:
• *Propranolol*
• *Cardiology consultation*
• *ICD placement*
• *Preoperative labs, including CBC, CMP, and coagulation profile*

Turn the clock forward, and the case will end. If the patient does poorly, order a surgical consult.

CASE 7: Acute Rheumatic Fever

Setting: *Office*

CC: *"My little boy has joint pain."*

Vitals: *Stable except for a temperature of 102°F*

HPI: *A 5-year-old boy presents with severe joint pain involving his knees, ankles, and wrists. He also complains of chest pain and shortness of breath, and his mother noticed a nonpruritic erythematous rash on his trunk, which has been enlarging. The child had a recent sore throat 2 weeks ago, but his mother doesn't believe in modern medicine and decided against antibiotics. The mother denies any recent travel history or insect bites.*

ROS: *No difficulty urinating*

Physical Exam:
- *Child appears to be having uncoordinated, rapid, jerking movements of the face, hands, and feet*
- *Macular erythematous rash on the trunk (Figure 10-6)*
- *Painful nodule on the wrists and elbows*
- *Tender joints to palpation in the knees and ankles*

Figure 10-6. Erythema marginatum of rheumatic fever. Enlarging and shifting transient annular and polycyclic lesions. (Reproduced with permission from Piette WW. Chapter 160. Rheumatoid arthritis, rheumatic fever, and gout. In: Goldsmith LA, et al., eds. *Fitzpatrick's Dermatology in General Medicine.* 8th ed. New York, NY: McGraw-Hill; 2012.)

What is the most likely diagnosis?

a. Kawasaki's disease

b. Rheumatic fever

c. Lyme disease

d. Septic arthritis

e. Reactive arthritis

Answer b. Rheumatic fever

Rheumatic fever is an inflammatory condition in which antibodies against streptococcus cross-reach with the heart and joints, producing symptoms such as carditis, polyarthritis, subcutaneous nodules, erythema marginatum, and Sydenham's chorea.

Kawasaki's disease is an inflammatory condition of the heart but would present with conjunctivitis, strawberry tongue, and a rash of the palms and soles. Lyme disease would have joint involvement but would have a history of insect bite or a rash known as erythema chronicum migrans. Septic arthritis would present with joint pain, but it would be one joint rather than multiple. Reactive arthritis presents after a recent infection, but it also presents with urethritis, which this patient does not have.

During a streptococcus infection, B cells present antigens to CD4-T cells, which differentiate into helper T_2 cells, which become plasma cells and produce antibodies. The antibodies cross-react against the myocardium and joints.

Acute rheumatic fever is the most common form acquired heart disease worldwide.

The most common bacteria to cause rheumatic fever is group A β-hemolytic streptococcal infection.

α-Hemolytic is green with partial hemolysis.
β-Hemolytic is clear with complete hemolysis.
γ-Hemolytic has no hemolysis.

What is the next best step in the management of this patient?

a. Antistreptolysin O (ASO) titer

b. Penicillin

c. Erythromycin

d. Chest radiography

e. ECG

Answer b. Penicillin

Penicillin for 10 days is the next best step in the management of this patient. There is no specific test to diagnose rheumatic fever, and the diagnosis of rheumatic fever can be made when two of the major criteria or one major criterion plus two minor criteria are met. Erythromycin is the drug of choice for patients who are allergic to penicillin. Chest radiography will show cardiomegaly but does not offer information to change the course of your management. ASO titers will be elevated, and ECG will show nonspecific findings, but neither of these is the next best step in the management of this patient.

ASO is used to detect streptococcal antibodies directed against streptococcal lysin O.

Modified Jones criteria: major criteria
   Joint (arthritis)
   Obvious (cardiac)
   Nodule (rheumatic)
   Erythema marginatum
   Sydenham's chorea

Jones criteria: minor criteria
   Inflammatory cells (leukocytosis)
   Temperature (fever)
   Elevated erythrocyte sedimentation rate or C-reactive protein
   Elevated PR interval
   Itself (previous history of rheumatic fever)
   Arthralgia

Aschoff bodies (Figure 10-7) are nodules found in patients with rheumatic fever and are composed of swollen eosinophilic collagen surrounded by lymphocytes and macrophages.

Orders:
• *Penicillin*
• *ECG*
• *Chest radiography*
• *ASO titer*
• *Infectious diseases consult*
• *Cardiology consult*

Turn the clock forward, and the case will end.

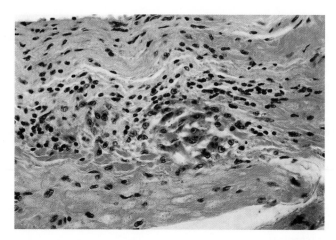

Figure 10-7. Reacting lymphocytes and large mononuclear cells in myocardium demonstrate a cellular component to the immune reaction in rheumatic fever. (Reproduced with permission from Ryan KJ, Ray C. Chapter 25. Streptococci and enterococci. In: Ryan KJ, Ray C, eds. *Sherris Medical Microbiology.* 5th ed. New York, NY: McGraw-Hill; 2010.)

> The most common ECG finding in patients with rheumatic fever is PR interval prolongation.

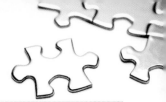

CHAPTER **11**

INFECTIOUS DISEASE

CASE 1: Red Eyes

Setting: *Ward*

CC: *"My child has red eyes."*

Vitals: *Stable*

HPI: *A newborn baby is brought in by his mother. His mother has just fed him. The mother noticed that the baby's eyes are very red, and she is concerned. She states that his delivery was uneventful even though she did not have any prenatal care.*

ROS:
• *No cough*
• *No coryza*

Physical Exam:
• *Scleral injection without discharge*

What is the most likely cause of conjunctivitis in a child younger than 24 hours of age?

a. Chemical conjunctivitis

b. Measles

c. Gonorrhea

d. Chlamydia

Answer a. Chemical conjunctivitis

The most common cause of conjunctivitis in a child younger than 24 hours is chemical conjunctivitis caused by eye drops placed by the delivery team to prevent infections. Typically at birth, a newborn baby is given two types of antibiotic drops in each eye to prevent infection later on. The most common ointments used are an erythromycin ointment, a tetracycline ointment, or a silver nitrate solution. The treatment for this form of conjunctivitis is supportive, and the condition is self-limited.

> Erythromycin is a bacteriostatic antibiotic that works by binding to the 50s subunit, thereby inhibiting protein synthesis by blocking translocation.

Tetracycline is an antibiotic that works binding to the 30s subunit, thereby inhibiting protein synthesis by blocking translocation.

Chemical irritation is typically caused by irritation from silver nitrate drops most commonly seen in developing countries; therefore, on your test, the USMLE will give clues such as that the patient is from an immigrant or uninsured family.

What is the most likely cause of conjunctivitis in a child who is 3 days old?

a. Chemical conjunctivitis

b. Measles

c. Gonorrhea

d. Chlamydia

Answer c. Gonorrhea

If the newborn presents with red, purulent eyes between day 2 and 7, the most likely agent is *Neisseria gonorrhea* as a cause of gonococcal ophthalmia neonatorum. *Neisseria* is gram-negative diplococci and is the primary reason prophylaxis ointments are provided at birth. A woman with a gonorrheal infection can easily pass the organism to her infant during birth, which can lead to a disseminated gonorrheal infection via infection in the conjunctiva.

Ceftriaxone inhibits bacterial cell wall synthesis by means of binding to the penicillin-binding proteins.

The incidence of gonococcal ophthalmia neonatorum has been dramatically reduced secondary to prophylaxis and is treated with ceftriaxone if an infection develops.

What is the most likely cause of conjunctivitis in a child who is 11 days old?

a. Herpes

b. Measles

c. Gonorrhea

d. Chlamydia

Answer d. Chlamydia

If the child had presented after 7 days, the most likely organism would be *Chlamydia trachomatis*.

The infection is treated with oral erythromycin. Even though erythromycin is the treatment of choice for chlamydial conjunctivitis, it is not effectively prevented by topical erythromycin at delivery.

Chlamydia trachomatis is an obligate intracellular human pathogen. Serotypes Ab, B, Ba, and C cause trachoma: infection of the eyes, which can lead to blindness

What is the most likely cause of conjunctivitis in a child who is 25 days old?

a. Herpes

b. Measles

c. Gonorrhea

d. Chlamydia

Answer a. Herpes

Conjunctivitis in a newborn older than 3 weeks old is most commonly secondary to herpes virus.

The infection is treated with acyclovir for approximately 10 to 14 days.

Acyclovir inhibits and inactivates HSV-specified DNA polymerases, preventing viral DNA synthesis.

CASE 2: Baby is Kind of Floppy

Setting: *ED*

CC: *"My baby is kind of floppy."*

Vitals: *Stable except for respiratory rate of 6*

HPI: *A 4-month-old baby girl is brought into the emergency department (ED) by her grandmother, who was watching the baby while her parents are away on vacation. The grandmother says the baby was in her usual state of health and playfulness, and when she began crying, the grandmother gave her some honey on her pacifier to sooth her. The grandmother noticed the baby became less playful and is now difficult to wake up.*

ROS:
- *No fevers*
- *No chills*
- *Normally fed by formula*

Physical Exam:
- *Not arousable*
- *Bluish tint to lips*
- *Hypotonia in all extremities (Figure 11-1)*
- *No meningeal signs*

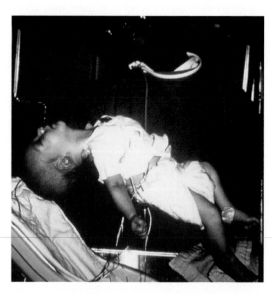

Figure 11-1. Infantile botulism. The floppy-constipated baby is a classic presentation of infantile botulism. (Reproduced with permission from Williams SR, Sztajnkrycer MD, Thurman R. Chapter 17. Toxicological conditions. In: Knoop KJ, Stack LB, Storrow AB, Thurman R, eds. *The Atlas of Emergency Medicine.* 3rd ed. New York, NY: McGraw-Hill; 2010.)

What is the most likely diagnosis?

a. Pneumonia

b. Botulism poisoning

c. Septic shock

d. Nonsteroidal antiinflammatory drug (NSAID) overdose

e. Meningitis

Answer b. Botulism poisoning

Botulinum poisoning presents in a child who is younger than 1 year of age who presents with severe hypotonia and respiratory paralysis after exposure to honey. It is caused by *Clostridium botulinum.* Pneumonia and septic shock would be in a patient with fever, and patients with meningitis have meningeal signs. NSAID overdoses would lead to metabolic complications and renal impairment.

> *C. botulinum* is an anaerobic, gram-positive, spore-forming rod.

> Eating honey during the first year of life has been identified as a risk factor for infant botulism.

What is the next best step in the management of this patient?

a. Intubation

b. Intravenous (IV) access

c. IV antibiotics

d. Check rectal temperature

e. Call intensive care unit (ICU) consult

Answer a. Intubation

The child is presenting with signs and symptoms of respiratory paralysis caused by botulinum toxin. The first step is to stabilize the child by intubating her and placing her on a ventilator followed by circulatory support with IV fluids. The other choices do not come before providing ventilator assistance.

> Botulinum toxin works by causing neuromuscular blockade through inhibition of acetylcholine's release from the presynaptic membrane of neuromuscular junctions in the somatic nervous system, leading to paralysis.

> Foodborne botulism results from contaminated food in which botulinum spores germinate and occurs in home-canned food most commonly.

What is the most appropriate therapy for a patient with botulinum poisoning?

a. Erythromycin   **c.** Antitoxin
b. Ampicillin   **d.** Supportive care and observation

Answer c. Antitoxin

The most appropriate treatment of botulism is with an antitoxin (human botulinum immunoglobulin) and supportive care.

Trivalent (A, B, E) botulinum antitoxin is derived from equine sources using whole antibodies. Heptavalent (A, B, C, D, E, F, G) botulinum antitoxin, which is derived from equine IgG antibodies.

A recommended preventive measure for infant botulism is to avoid giving honey to infants younger than 12 months of age. Prevention is the best therapy because there is no vaccine.

Orders:
• Botulinum antitoxin
• Admit to the ICU

CASE 3: Bad Kitty

Setting: *Office*

CC: *"My kid got scratched."*

Vitals: *Stable except for fever of 101.1°F*

HPI: *A 5-year-old girl presents with fevers. The child's mother noted that the child has had high fevers and swelling in the neck and underarm area. The child also complaints of joint pains, backache, chills, and abdominal pain. The mother mentions she has to go home and feed their new kitten.*

ROS:
- *No nausea*
- *No vomiting*

Physical Exam:
- *Tender lymphadenopathy in the axilla*
- *Scratches on the hands bilaterally*

What is the most likely organism to cause this diagnosis?

a. Cat scratch
b. Cat bite

c. Dog bite
d. Human bite

Answer a. Cat scratch

The patient presents with cat scratch disease (CSD) caused by *Bartonella henselae.* It commonly presents 1 to 2 weeks after a kitten scratches a child and presents with lymphadenopathy, joint pains, and high fevers. The patients can also have systemic effects such as arthralgias, abdominal pain, and malaise. Cat and dog bites can lead to infection with *Pasturella multocida,* and human bites can lead to *Eikenella* infections.

B. henselae is gram-negative bacillus with a polar flagellum.

What is the next best step in the management of this patient?

a. Observation
b. Azithromycin

c. Rifampin
d. Erythromycin

Answer a. Observation

Virtually all cases of CSD remit spontaneously without therapeutic intervention. Antibiotics such as azithromycin are only recommended for immunocompromised patients.

The Warthin-Starry stain shows the presence of *B. henselae* but is not necessary because the diagnosis can be made clinically.

The most accurate diagnostic test is polymerase chain reaction, but it is only needed if the patient's diagnosis is equivocal.

Orders:
• *Send the patient home and bring her back in 2 weeks.*

CASE 4: Spots

Setting: *Office*

CC: *"My child is covered in spots."*

Vitals: *Fever of 102.5°F*

HPI: *A mother presents to the ED with her 3-year-old daughter. The mother and daughter are both from South America. The mother is unaware of what immunizations the little girl has, if any. A rash was noted that began on the back of the head and neck and is starting working its way down to the trunk. The mother also says the child's eyes have been red.*

ROS:
- *Cough*
- *Nasal congestion*

Physical Exam:
- *Severe conjunctivitis of both eyes*
- *Generalized, maculopapular, erythematous rash (Figure 11-2)*
- *Grayish white dots are seen on the buccal mucosa next to the third molar (Figure 11-3)*

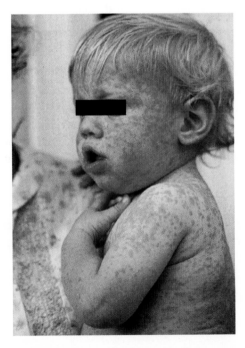

Figure 11-2. Measles rash on day 4 of illness. (Reproduced with permission from Ryan KJ, Ray C. Chapter 10. Viruses of mumps, measles, rubella, and other childhood exanthems. In: Ryan KJ, Ray C, eds. *Sherris Medical Microbiology.* 6th ed. New York, NY: McGraw-Hill; 2014.)

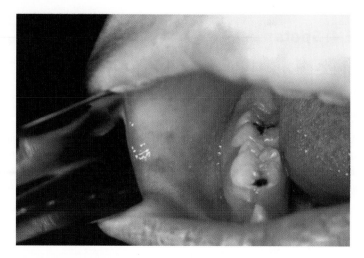

Figure 11-3. Koplik spots. (Reproduced with permission from Bonfante G, Rosenau AM. Chapter 134. Rashes in infants and children. In: Tintinalli JE, et al., eds. *Tintinalli's Emergency Medicine: A Comprehensive Study Guide.* 7th ed. New York, NY: McGraw-Hill; 2011.)

What is the most likely diagnosis?

a. Measles

b. Rubella

c. Roseola

d. Mumps

e. Varicella

Answer a. Measles

Measles is a viral illness that occurs in young children who are unvaccinated against the disease. It classically presents with a rash that begins on the head and spreads down to the trunk. The prodrome of the illness includes a cough, coryza, conjunctivitis, and then Koplik spots (grayish spots on the buccal mucosa). Rubella is a rash that begins on the face, roseola has a rash that is seen on the third or fourth day after fever, and mumps would have orchitis and parotitis.

Measles virus is a single-stranded, negative-sense, enveloped RNA virus of the genus *Morbillivirus* within the family Paramyxoviridae.

Measles = the 4 Cs
- Cough
- Coryza
- Conjunctivitis
- Koplik spots

What is the next best step in management?

a. Measles titers

b. Observation

c. Vitamin A

d. IV fluids

e. Measles, mumps, and rubella (MMR) vaccination

Answer b. Observation

The diagnosis and treatment of measles include observation and supportive treatment. There is no specific treatment for measles. Most patients with uncomplicated measles recover with rest and supportive treatment. Vitamin A has no role in the treatment of measles and is the most common wrong answer. Measles titers take too long, and the diagnosis can be made through clinical exam.

Subacute sclerosing panencephalitis is gradual, progressive encephalitis, consisting of personality change, seizures, and myoclonus caused by persistent measles virus. It is a USMLE favorite.

The best form of treatment for measles is prevention.

Orders:
• *Send the patient home and bring her back in 2 weeks.*

The most common complication of measles is otitis media.

CASE 5: Three-Day Measles

Setting: *Office*

CC: *"My child has a rash . . . can we hurry this up?"*

Vitals: *Stable except for fever of 102°F*

HPI: *A 5-year-old child with an absentee mother and known noncompliance with immunizations presents to the office. The child has been feeling unwell. His rash began his face and spread to the rest of his body. The mother says the rash occurred at the same time her son felt warm.*

Physical Exam:
- *Pinpoint rash* (Figure 11-4)
- *Postoccipital and retroauricular lymphadenopathy*
- *Rose spots on the soft palate*

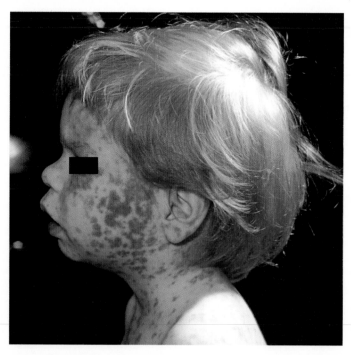

Figure 11-4. Rubella. (Reproduced with permission from Bonfante G, Rosenau AM. Chapter 134. Rashes in infants and children. In: Tintinalli JE, et al., eds. *Tintinalli's Emergency Medicine: A Comprehensive Study Guide.* 7th ed. New York, NY: McGraw-Hill; 2011.)

What is the most likely diagnosis?

a. Measles

b. Rubella

c. Roseola

d. Mumps

e. Varicella

Answer b. Rubella

Rubella presents similar to measles in that a rash occurs, but it starts on the face and then spreads to the rest of the body. It occurs concurrently with a fever and has lymphadenopathy in the postoccipital, retroauricular, and occiput. Measles would have a rash that starts at the head and moves down, and roseola is a rash that follows the fever. Varicella would not be a maculopapular rash but would be vesicular.

> Forschheimer spots are rose spots that are seen on the soft palate before the rash.

> Rubella virus is a togavirus that is enveloped and has a single-stranded RNA genome.

> The diagnosis of rubella is made by clinical diagnosis.

> On the USMLE, all viral exanthems are based on the timing of the fever and the appearance of the rash.

What is the most appropriate therapy for this patient?

a. Observation

b. Antipyretics

c. Topical steroids

d. Oral rehydration

Answer a. Observation

There is no specific treatment for rubella except for observation and supportive care of symptoms. Antipyretics alone are not the best therapy, topical steroids have no therapy, and oral rehydration is only indicated if the child has symptoms of dehydration.

> HLA-A1 genotypes are associated with increased susceptibility to infection.

Rubella as a TORCH infection
• Patent ductus arteriosus is the most common finding
• Blindness
• Deafness
• "Blueberry muffin" skin rash

Orders: *Send the patient home and bring him back in 2 weeks.*

CASE 6: Fever First, Rash Later

Setting: *Office*

CC: *"My baby has a rash."*

Vitals: *Stable*

HPI: *An 18-month-old girl is brought to her pediatrician's office because of a rash that appeared today. The baby has had a fever for the past 3 days. The fever is gone today, but the rash is all over her body. The rash appears pink and is raised. Her mother is very concerned and wants to know what do.*

Physical Exam:
* *Rose-colored maculopapular rash over the entire body (Figure 11-5)*

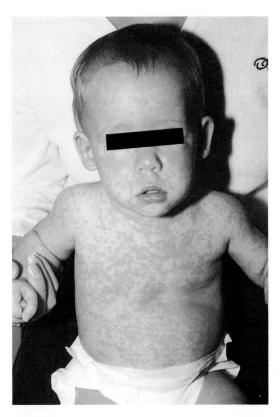

Figure 11-5. Roseola infantum. (Reproduced with permission from Roseola infantum. Bonfante G, Rosenau AM. Chapter 134. Rashes in infants and children. In: Tintinalli JE, et al., eds. *Tintinalli's Emergency Medicine: A Comprehensive Study Guide.* 7th ed. New York, NY: McGraw-Hill; 2011.)

What is the most likely diagnosis?

a. Measles

b. Rubella

c. Roseola

d. Mumps

Answer c. Roseola

Roseola is a febrile illness of viral etiology caused by a human herpes virus 6 (HHV-6) infection. It is most common in children younger than 5 years of age. The clinical presentation of a fever and most commonly presents as a fever for 3 or 4 days followed by a rose-colored maculopapular rash. It is collectively caused sixth's disease.

The diagnosis of roseola is based on clinical diagnosis; the treatment is supportive.

Roseola is caused by human herpes viruses HHV-6, which is sometimes referred to collectively as Roseolovirus.

Orders:

• *Send the patient home and bring her back in 2 weeks.*

• *Acetaminophen*

CASE 7: Mumps

Setting: *Office*

CC: *"My child's face is swollen, and he has a fever."*

Vitals: *Stable except for fever of 102.8°F*

HPI: *A 3-year-old boy is brought to the clinic by his mother for swelling in his face and fever that has lasted for the last 5 days. He has never had vaccinations because his parents were afraid of side effects.*

Physical Exam:
- *Bilateral facial swelling near the masseter and angle of the mandible*
- *Swollen testicles*
- *Epigastric tenderness*

What is the most likely diagnosis?

a. Measles

b. Rubella

c. Roseola

d. Mumps

Answer d. Mumps

Mumps is a viral infection caused by a paramyxovirus and presents with fevers, bilateral parotid gland enlargement, and possibly orchitis or pancreatitis. This is a viral syndrome without any rash.

Orchitis or oophoritis + Pancreatitis + Parotiditis = Mumps

The most common risk factor for mumps is missed vaccinations.

What is the most common complication of mumps?

a. Sterility

b. Meningoencephalomyelitis

c. Myocarditis

d. Deafness

e. Pancreatitis

Answer b. Meningoencephalomyelitis

Meningoencephalomyelitis is the most common complication of having mumps. Sterility is the most common wrong answer and only occurs if orchitis is bilateral. The diagnosis of mumps is a clinical diagnosis, and the treatment is supportive.

Acetaminophen is used over aspirin because of the risk of Reye's syndrome.

Patients are contagious 1 day before and 3 days after the swelling appears.

Orders:
• *Send the patient home and bring him back in 2 weeks.*
• *Acetaminophen*

CASE 8: Fifths, Not Sixths

Setting: *Office*

CC: *"I think the babysitter slapped my daughter's face."*

Vitals: *Stable except for fever 101.5°F*

HPI: *A 5-year-old girl is bought into the doctor's office. The mother is worried that her babysitter slapped the baby across both her cheeks. She is concerned about the red marks on her cheeks. The girl also has a lacy rash across the upper extremities and trunk. The mother states it has been there for about 5 days.*

Physical Exam:
- *A red rash on the cheeks*
- *Lacy lenticular rash on the upper arms, torso, and legs (Figure 11-6)*
- *Sparing of the palm and soles*
- *Pain with palpation of the hips and elbows*

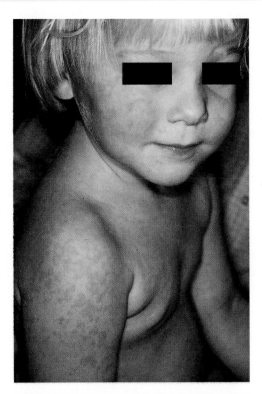

Figure 11-6. Erythema infectiosum (fifth disease). (Reproduced with permission from Erythema infectiosum (Fifth disease). Bonfante G, Rosenau AM. Chapter 134. Rashes in infants and children. In: Tintinalli JE, et al., eds. *Tintinalli's Emergency Medicine: A Comprehensive Study Guide.* 7th ed. New York, NY: McGraw-Hill; 2011.)

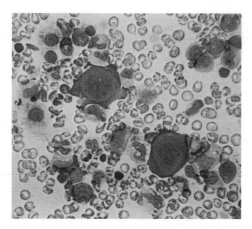

Figure 11-7. Pathognomonic cells in marrow failure syndromes. Giant pronormoblast, the cytopathic effect of B19 parvovirus infection of the erythroid progenitor cell. (Reproduced with permission from Young NS. Chapter 107. Aplastic anemia, myelodysplasia, and related bone marrow failure syndromes. In: Longo DL, et al., eds. *Harrison's Principles of Internal Medicine*. 18th ed. New York, NY: McGraw-Hill; 2012.)

What is the most likely diagnosis?

a. Varicella   **d.** Mumps

b. Erythema infectiosum   **e.** Measles

c. Rubella

Answer b. Erythema infectiosum

Erythema infectiosum is a viral exanthem secondary to a parvovirus B19 infection (Figure 11-7). The child will present with a very red "slapped cheek" look with a reticular rash on the extremities and sparing of the palms and soles. The rash may be present for up to 40 days. Varicella would have vesicles, and measles, mumps, and rubella present with a rash but do not have an intensely slapped cheek appearance. The diagnosis of the syndrome is based on clinical findings, and the treatment is supportive with antipyretics.

> Parvovirus B19 is a nonenveloped, icosahedral virus that contains a single-stranded linear DNA genome.

Order:
• *Send the patient as the infection will self-resolve.*

> The diagnosis of parvovirus B19 is a clinical diagnosis, and the disease is self-limiting. The treatment is supportive observation.

Parvovirus B19 + Pregnant women = Hydrops fetalis causing spontaneous miscarriage

Parvovirus B19 + Sickle cell disease = Aplastic crisis

Parvovirus B19 + HIV/AIDS = Infection

CASE 9: Scarlet Fever

Setting: *ED*

CC: *"My child's tongue is swollen."*

Vitals: *Stable except for fever*

HPI: *A 7-year-old boy is brought into the ED by his father after he notices his son's tongue is beefy and swollen. The child has been complaining of a sore throat for the past few days, and the father recently noticed the child had a rash.*

ROS:
• *Pain with swallowing*

Physical Exam:
• *"Strawberry" appearance to the tongue (*Figure 11-8*)*
• *Forchheimer spots*
• *Fine, red, rough-textured rash that blanches with pressure*
• *Peeling of the skin on the palms and soles*

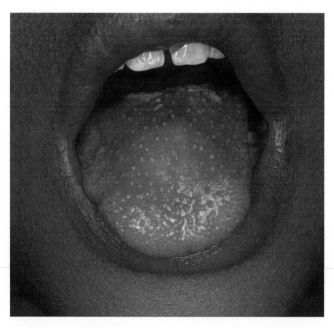

Figure 11-8. Strawberry tongue. This patient with scarlet fever demonstrates the bright red appearance of strawberry tongue after most of the white exudate is lost. (Reproduced with permission from Jauch EC, Gottesman BE. Chapter 6. Mouth. In: Knoop KJ, Stack LB, Storrow AB, Thurman R, eds. *The Atlas of Emergency Medicine.* 3rd ed. New York, NY: McGraw-Hill; 2010.)

What is the most likely diagnosis?

a. Scarlet fever

b. Roseola

c. Varicella

d. Measles

e. Rubella

Answer a. Scarlet fever

Scarlet fever is an infectious disease caused by *Streptococcus pyogenes* that presents with a sore throat, strawberry tongue, and sandpaper-like rash that blanches easily. The rashes in the inguinal areas and folds of the body are very red (known as Pastia lines). The other disorders have no tongue involvement; there are very few things in medicine that make a person's tongue look like a strawberry. Kawasaki's disease has a strawberry tongue but also has uveitis, conjunctival inflammation, and lymphadenopathy.

An erythrogenic toxin is a toxin produced by strains of *S. pyogenes*, the primary cause of scarlet fever.

S. pyogenes is a spherical, gram-positive organism that is also known as group A (β-hemolytic) streptococcus.

What is the next best step in the management of this patient?

a. Complete blood count

b. Erythrocyte sedimentation rate

c. Antistreptolysin O (ASO) titers

d. Antipyretics

e. Penicillin

Answer e. Penicillin

Penicillin is the next best step in the management of this patient. The diagnosis of scarlet fever is made clinically though history and physical findings. Streptococcal antibody tests such as ASO titers are used to confirm previous group A streptococcal infection, but the titer may not be elevated early in the infection.

ASO is an antibody that is produced when the body is infected with streptococci, which later cross-reacts with human collagen in the heart and joints.

Erythromycin is considered the alternative for penicillin-allergic patients.

The most common complications are acute rheumatic fever and glomerulonephritis.

Orders:
- *Penicillin*
- *Follow-up appointment in 2 to 4 weeks*

CASE 10: **Whoop, There It Is**

Setting: *ED*

CC: *"My child wont stop coughing."*

Vitals: *HR, 101 beats/min; BP, 120/78 mm Hg; RR, 24 breaths/min; afebrile*

HPI: *An 8-year-old boy is brought to the ED for coughing. His mother says he has a cough that will not go away that has lasted 15 days or longer. In the ED, the child is coughing repeatedly, and after several episodes of coughing, he gasps loudly for air. The child has been going to daycare, and the mother states she does not believe in vaccinating her child because she will not be told how to raise her baby.*

PMH:
• *Macrocytic anemia from lack of vitamin B$_{12}$ caused by a vegan diet*

ROS:
• *Vomiting after extreme episodes of coughing*
• *Recent upper respiratory infection*
• *Runny nose, sneezing, and low-grade fever*

Physical Exam:
• *Conjunctival hemorrhage of the left eye*
• *Facial petechiae*

What is the most likely diagnosis?

a. *Bordetella pertussis*
b. Croup
c. Epiglottitis

d. Pneumonia
e. Upper respiratory infection

Answer a. *Bordetella pertussis*

B. pertussis is a infection of the upper respiratory tract in which there are three phases; it is characterized by fits of coughing followed by gasping for air, which sounds like a large whoop. The most common risk factor is being unvaccinated to DTap (diphtheria, tetanus, and pertussis). Croup would present with upper airway narrowing and stridor, and epiglottitis causes tripoding, drooling, and high fevers. Pneumonia would present with fevers, coughing, and sputum with a consolidation on chest radiography.

B. pertussis ADP ribosylates GI (inhibitor), reducing its responsiveness to the receptor, thus increasing cAMP.

B. *pertussis* is a gram-negative, aerobic coccobacillus that grows on Bordet-Gengou agar.

Pertussis vaccine is part of the DTap injection.

What are the three stages of pertussis in order?

a. Catarrhal, paroxysmal, convalescent
b. Paroxysmal, convalescent, catarrhal
c. Convalescent, paroxysmal, catarrhal
d. None of the above

Answer a. Catarrhal, paroxysmal, convalescent

The catarrhal phase is the first 2 weeks and presents with coldlike symptoms such as cough, rhinorrhea, and conjunctival injection. The paroxysmal phase lasts for 2 to 5 weeks and presents with coughing fits followed by a whooping inspiratory sound. The convalescent phase lasts more than 2 weeks and is basic resolution of cough.

What is the most appropriate diagnostic test?

a. Azithromycin
b. Supportive care
c. Treat household members
d. Polymerase chain reaction (PCR) assay for *B. pertussis*
e. All of the above

Answer d. Polymerase chain reaction (PCR) assay for *B. pertussis*

An acute coughing illness that lasts at least 14 days in a person with at least one characteristic pertussis symptom such as a whooping cough should be treated with azithromycin and supportive care. A PCR assay should be performed but *should not* delay treatment. The physician should treat first and follow up with the PCR afterward.

Close household contacts should receive 5 days of azithromycin.

Diphtheria toxin, *Pseudomonas* exotoxin, *Escherichia coli* heat-labile toxin, cholera toxin, and pertussis toxin are the ADP-ribosylating toxins.

Orders:

• *Azithromycin*

Change the location to floors. Turn to the clock to the next morning for rounds, and the case will end.

CASE 11: Steeples and Coughs

Setting: *ED*

CC: *"My child is not breathing well."*

Vitals: *Stable*

HPI: *A 3-year-old child is brought to the ED for a persistent cough. The mother states that her child has a cough that scares their dog because it sounds like barking. Chest radiography shows a narrowing of the upper airway without foreign body.*

ROS:
• *Hoarseness*

Physical Exam:
• *Barking cough*
• *Inspiratory stridor*
• *No cyanosis*

What is the most likely diagnosis?

a. Croup

b. Epiglottitis

c. Pertussis

d. Foreign body

Answer a. Croup

Croup is a viral infection of the upper airway that causes white blood cell infiltration and swelling of the upper neck. The cough is characterized by inspiratory stridor and a barking cough. The most accurate test is a PCR for virus, but it is not needed clinically. Epiglottis is difficulty swallowing and drooling, and a foreign body would be seen on radiography.

> The steeple sign is seen on a neck radiography of a child with croup (Figure 11-9).

> The most common causes of viral croup are parainfluenza virus types 1 and 2.

What is the most appropriate therapy for croup?

a. Nebulized epinephrine

b. Single-dose dexamethasone

c. Supportive care

d. Intubation

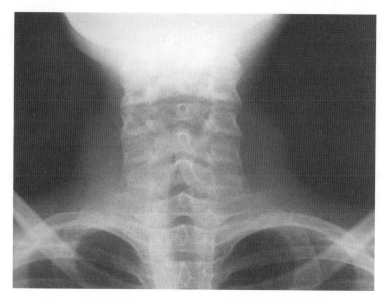

Figure 11-9. Steeple sign. (Reproduced with permission from Stallard TC. Chapter 32. Emergency disorders of the ear, nose, sinuses, oropharynx, & mouth. In: Stone C, Humphries RL, eds. *CURRENT Diagnosis & Treatment Emergency Medicine.* 7th ed. New York, NY: McGraw-Hill; 2011.)

Answer b. Single-dose dexamethasone

The most appropriate therapy is single-dose dexamethasone. Intubation and nebulized epinephrine are the appropriate therapy if the child has severe disease characterized by cyanosis and findings of both inspiratory expiratory stridor with progressing to stridor at rest.

> If gray membranes are seen in the posterior pharynx, then *Corynebacterium diphtheriae* is likely the most common cause.

Orders:
- *Dexamethasone*
- *Admit to the ICU*

CASE 12: **Drool Everywhere**

Setting: *ED*

CC: *"My child cannot swallow."*

Vitals: *Stable except for fever of 102.9°F*

HPI: *A 6-year-old boy presents with a sudden onset of an extremely sore throat and high fevers and is drooling and cannot tolerate his secretions.*

ROS:
- *High fever at home*
- *Cannot swallow*
- *Cannot talk*

Physical Exam:
- *Stridor heard on passive breathing*
- *Hot potato voice*
- *Tripoding position*

What is the most likely diagnosis?

a. Croup

b. Epiglottitis

c. Pertussis

d. Foreign body

Answer b. Epiglottitis

Epiglottitis is an inflammatory process of the epiglottis caused by the bacterium *Haemophilus influenzae* type B. The epiglottis becomes swollen and subsequently causes fever, difficulty in swallowing, and drooling. As the swelling worsens, hoarseness of the voice and stridor develop. The child will present with tripodding to allow the salvia to drip out of his mouth because he is unable to tolerate his secretions.

Epiglottitis is due to a bacterial infection of the epiglottis, most often caused by *Haemophilus influenzae* type B.

The most common causes of epiglottitis in immunocompromised patients are Candida and Aspergillus spp.

The most common cause of epiglottitis in adults is thermal injury caused by smoking crack cocaine.

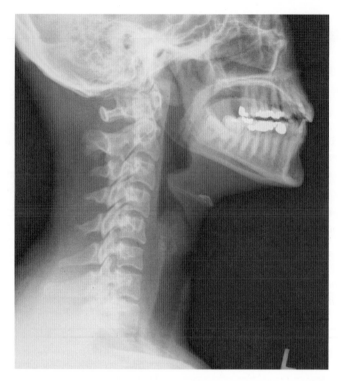

Figure 11-10. Adult Epiglottitis. Soft-tissue lateral neck radiograph of an adult with epiglottitis demonstrating the classic "thumb" sign of a swollen epiglottis. (Reproduced with permission from Jauch EC, et al. Chapter 5. Ear, nose, and throat conditions. In: Knoop KJ, Stack LB, Storrow AB, Thurman R, eds. *The Atlas of Emergency Medicine.* 3rd ed. New York, NY: McGraw-Hill; 2010.)

What is the most common finding on neck radiography?

a. Thumbprint sign

b. Elbow sign

c. Steeple sign

d. Fischer sign

e. Bird's beak sign

Answer a. Thumbprint sign

The most common finding on a patient with epiglottitis is a thumbprint sign (Figure 11-10), which is seen on a lateral cervical spine radiograph. The thumbprint actually denotes a swollen and enlarged epiglottis with a dilated hypopharynx.

The best initial test for diagnosing epiglottitis is an radiography, but the most accurate test is direct visualization of the epiglottis using nasopharyngoscopy or laryngoscopy, neither of which should occur without securing an airway.

What is the next best step in the management of this patient?

a. Racemic epinephrine

b. Intubation in the ED

c. Intubation in the operating room (OR)

d. Observation

e. Steroids

f. Antibiotics

Answer c. Intubation in the operating room (OR)

The most urgent issue in a patient with epiglottitis is airway management because the slightest irritation or manipulation of the epiglottis could result in complete airway closure; therefore, intubation in a monitored setting is the best next step in management. If oral intubation fails or the airway closes off, a surgical airway procedure known as a cricothyrotomy must be performed, thus the reason for having it take place in the OR. Radiologic testing, antibiotics, and other testing are all secondary to obtaining a patent airway.

Racemic epinephrine, corticosteroids, and β-agonists have not been proven to be helpful in epiglottitis.

Third-generation cephalosporins such as ceftriaxone are the drugs of choice for epiglottitis.

Orders:

- *Intubation*
- *Anesthesia consult for intubation*
- *Ear, nose, and throat consult for possible laryngoscopy*
- *Lateral neck radiography after intubation*
- *Ceftriaxone*
- *Acetaminophen*

Turn the clock forward and transfer the patient to the ICU.

INDEX

Page numbers followed by *f* or *t* indicate figures or tables, respectively.